WE ARE NOT ALONE

Learning to Live with Chronic Illness

SEFRA
KOBRIN
PITZELE

*Illustrations by
Michael J. Fornwald*

Workman Publishing • New York

Library of Congress Cataloging-in-Publication Data

Pitzele, Sefra, 1942–
We are not alone.

Bibliography: p.
Includes index.
1. Chronic diseases—Psychological aspects.
2. Chronically ill—Family relationships. I. Title.
RC108.P57   1986   362.1'9   86-40200
ISBN 0-89480-139-2 (pbk.)

The recipes on pages 247 to 250 are from
The *American Heart Association Cookbook,* Copyright © 1984,
and reprinted with permission granted
by David McKay Company, Inc.

Art director: Charles Kreloff
Book design: Linda Peterson
Cover photograph: Jila Nikpay

First published in June 1985 by Thompson & Company, Inc.

Workman Publishing
1 West 39 Street
New York, New York 10018

Manufactured in the United States of America
First Workman printing September 1986

10 9 8 7 6 5 4 3 2 1

ACKNOWLEDGMENTS

This book is gratefully dedicated to everyone who has reached out to help another person. I want to extend a special thank you to the following groups and individuals:

To my children, Debbi, Mark, and Amy, who have matured so rapidly because of my illness.

To Chuck, who has struggled to make his own adjustment.

To my friends, who were there when I needed them. Thank you for helping me to begin again.

To my personal physician and friend, Dr. Thomas Reid Smith, who has listened, understood, and treated me with expertise and deep caring. You are the kind of physician all patients should be privileged to have treat them at least once in their lifetime.

To Dr. Judith Steller, a psychologist and friend who specializes in coping, for being "the glue that held me together" during these many months of illness and continuing adjustment.

To Dr. Paul Waytz, my rheumatologist, for your expertise and patient explanations.

To Brad Thompson and Anne Carroll at Thompson & Company, my editors and friends, for their faith, ability, and caring.

Finally, I want to thank the literally hundreds of people at associations for the ill who offered continued encouragement and support. I don't know all of your names, but your collective efforts make all the difference to those of us who call on you for help.

—Sefra Kobrin Pitzele
St. Paul, Minnesota

CONTENTS

INTRODUCTION

*C*hronic illness is on the increase.

Modern medical technologies have led to earlier detection, intervention and control of *acute* illness, and consequently, we will all live longer. Longevity increases the probability of developing a chronic illness, as well as acquiring the "aches and pains" previously ascribed solely to the aging process. Getting old in America very often means learning to live with a chronic illness, disability, or condition for the remainder of your life.

For at least the past generation, our society has romanticized and revered standards of health and fitness to the exclusion of the less healthy and the less fit. Unfortunately, the reality of chronic illness has been neglected.

Approximately 30 percent of our adult population suffers from a chronic illness. More than 50 million Americans now suffer from one of the "dirty dozen" most common chronic illnesses that are the focus of *We Are Not Alone:*

1. Rheumatoid arthritis
2. Ankylosing spondylitis
3. All other related arthritic illnesses
4. Systemic lupus erythematosus
5. Parkinson's disease
6. Emphysema
7. Multiple sclerosis
8. Heart disease
9. Stroke with permanent impairment
10. Asthma severe enough to impair
11. Dystrophies severe enough to impair
12. Diabetes

While these illnesses are medically distinct, the effect upon their victims is similar. A chronic illness is:

■ Permanent

■ The cause of frequent and costly medical intervention

■ The cause of substantial modification of—
Lifestyle
Life goals
Vocational choices and opportunities
Recreational activities
Interpersonal relationships
Family role or position

Chronic illness also presents a continuous series of unfamiliar stresses and challenges which require adjustments that were previously unnecessary and unknown.

As a psychiatrist who has specialized in the problems of the chronically ill and handicapped, I've become accustomed to the monumental psychological trauma experienced by the newly diagnosed victim of a chronic illness or handicap. I am regularly impressed with the resilience of the human spirit as people cope with the inevitable sequence of psychological adjustments: Initial denial, shock, depression, regression, perhaps despair, gradual acceptance, and adjustment.

The common attribute shared by those who are newly diagnosed with a chronic illness is *their lack of preparedness for the adaptations and adjustments dictated by their specific illness.* Commonplace in the newly diagnosed patient is an enormous craving for a reliable guide to their condition written in clear, accurate, sensible, compassionate, and practical terms. Rarely are physicians accessible enough to satisfy the patient's emotional need for reassurance and to answer the countless questions.

What has been needed is a book such as *We Are Not Alone.* The author, Sefra Pitzele, writes with much compassion and insight gleaned from her personal battle with her chronic illnesses, systemic lupus erythematosus and Sjogren's Syndrome.

We Are Not Alone is a masterfully written book, full of wisdom and practical guidance. It is unique in its presentation of the emotional and mental rigors of coping with a chronic illness, and it offers new insights into the stages of change, the stress of new communication patterns, and the process of readjustment.

This hopeful, comprehensive guide for the patient and his or her family covers all phases of chronic illness, from the frightening and uncertain prediagnosis stage, through the state of lost health, vigor, independence, and autonomy, through the changes in self-image and self-esteem, all the way to the ticklish issues of dealing with relationships. Of particular value are the sections on explaining your chronic illness to your spouse and children. I believe you will find the material that addresses the patient's relationship with his or her doctor critically important to the successful management of your illness.

Other topics that are especially useful include the issues of patienthood, self-monitoring, adaptive living strategies, and where-to-find-the-right-kind-of-help resources. This book is a powerful networking tool that lists resource groups, patient advocate and support organizations (including descriptions, addresses and phone numbers), and reviews of available materials.

I found this to be an uplifting book. Not only does the author confront the realities of living with chronic illness, but because she also provides badly needed information, she offers hope. As she appraises the process of adaptation through the seasoned eyes of a person who suffers herself, the reader gains an appreciation for how great the personal struggles and the victories are.

I know of no other book on this topic that can be as useful a tool as this. I know of no other book that can directly guide the patient and his or her family toward an acceptable adaptation to a chronic illness.

My one regret is that this compelling and inspirational manuscript was not available to me some 15 years ago when I became chronically ill with a connective tissue disease. It would have made my personal road to adaptation shorter and a little easier to travel. It is my sincere wish that the reader find peace and answers here.

—Howard Steven Shapiro, M.D., Assistant Clinical Professor of Psychiatry and Behavioral Sciences, University of Southern California School of Medicine and Medical Advisor to the Greater Los Angeles Chapter of the Lupus Foundation of America

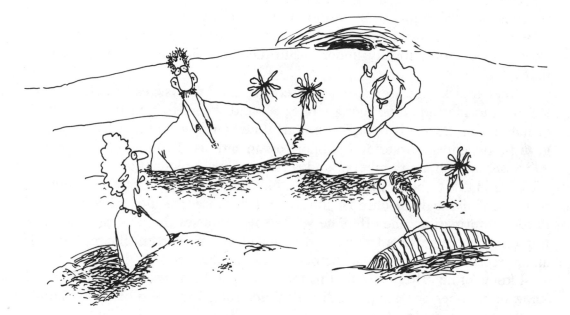

Chronic illnesses are like dandelions. You never know where they will pop up.

WHO PROMISED LIFE WOULD ALWAYS BE FAIR?

*I*t didn't take me long to realize that I wasn't going to be one of the exceptional few to recover from a chronic illness. Despite my optimism and resolve, I was humbled every day by reminders that my body was a traitor to my physical and mental well-being. If you, too, understand this experience, you will find this book helpful.

This book is about learning to live with a chronic illness or a chronic medical condition. It is the story each one of us can tell about the unpredictable, frightening, and maddening parts of living with a chronic illness. Mostly, it is the story of how to find a new lifestyle and a new definition of "normal."

Only a small part of this book is about me. Most of it is for and about *us*. I wrote it also for our families and friends who are unwilling witnesses to our frustrations and our greatest allies in our fight to live as normally as possible.

If you haven't heard it yet, let me be the one to tell you the truth: Chronic illness is forever. It hurts. It's lousy and unfair. You are going to have to learn to cope with your illness or condition, and you are going to have to keep at it for the rest of your life. Your struggle will probably get harder before it gets easier. It is very doubtful that there is or will be a miracle cure that restores you to your desired level of vitality and strength. Your life is going to be different from now on; you have suffered a permanent change.

You and I are not alone. Many, many people suffer from chronic illnesses. According to 1985 estimates by associations and research foundations organized to help us, one-third of the adult population in America—over 55 million people—suffer from diseases like these:

Arthritic Diseases:
- *Rheumatoid arthritis* *16,000,000*
- *Osteoarthritis* *16,000,000*
- *Gout.* *1,800,000*
- *Ankylosing spondylitis.* *2,500,000*
- *Other arthritic diseases* *4,000,000*
- *Systemic lupus erythematosus* *500,000*
- *Parkinson's disease* *1,500,000*
- *Multiple sclerosis* *250,000*
- *Lung disease severe enough to impair* *3,169,000*
- *Heart disease with permanent impairment* *4,600,000*
- *Stroke with permanent impairment.* *1,870,000*
- *Adult-onset dystrophies.* *200,000*
- *Diabetes Type I (insulin dependent)* *500,000*
- *Diabetes Type II (non-insulin dependent)* *5,000,000*

These statistics do *not* include undiagnosed and unreported sufferers, who nevertheless feel real symptoms. Furthermore, these statistics do not count those who are afflicted with cancer, other coronary diseases, discoid lupus, rheumatic heart disease, other progressive neuro-muscular diseases, or any other chronic condition that has radically altered their way of life. For every man like my father, who had Parkinson's disease, there are thousands more who suspect there is a problem but who are afraid to ask. They are not counted as statistics, either.

Nor do these statistics reflect the anguish and frustration of the friends and families close to each of the afflicted listed above. A census of the chronically ill does not count the tears shed in shame and anger, and it does not even begin to measure the effect of our fears.

You and I are not alone. We are all doing our best to get through one day at a time, hoping for a remission or change that will lighten our burdens, however temporarily. We share the uncertain, shadow-laden lives of the chronically ill that lurk behind the statistics. We share the same fear of not being able to support our families. We share the same depression and despair as we feel our lives slip away from us, out of our control. Our plans, our dreams, our quality of life—they all seem to be rolling downhill, faster and faster. At one time or another, we all grow exhausted trying vainly to halt and reverse the inevitable changes brought on by our illness.

The symptoms of my disease may differ from yours, and I may be listed on a different row in the statistics, but you and I and the other readers of this book have much in common. We share the crushing loneliness. We wonder why we were singled out for illness. And, occasionally, we let self-pity overwhelm us.

I have passed through the same hell you have, and still fight every day against my symptoms to achieve a higher quality of life. I want to share with you what I and others have learned.

Knowing that others suffer with us does not lessen our pain. But we *can* learn from each other. Each of us has learned valuable lessons that can help someone else. We all belong to the "community" of the chronically ill, and we can help each other cope by sharing what we have learned. This book is my modest contribution to that effort, representing my experiences and those of many others I have had the privilege to meet.

---

66 Some people have only learned 'to put up with' their problems. They may have given up hope. We need to tell them and show them that there is still much happiness and dignity and love to fight for. **99**

——SEFRA PITZELE

True, our lives have changed, probably forever. But weren't they going to change sooner or later anyway? Is it possible that, in many respects, our illnesses are similar to other events that naturally occur, such as career changes, the death of a parent or spouse, an unplanned job transfer, a legal problem, retirement, sexual difficulties, or a significant change in our financial situation? Someday, one way or the other, we would—and perhaps will—have to cope with these changes, too.

We are different from other people now. Chronic illness has changed our lives forever, and we are going to have to accept change routinely from now on. Some changes will be profound; many will be minor. How well we accept the consequences of our conditions and how well we adapt to the changes will determine how happy and satisfying the rest of our lives will be.

> **"** We can't say this any more: 'Everything else may be going wrong, but at least I still have my health!' It's no longer true. Now, all we can say is, 'It could be a lot worse.' **"**
>
> —SEFRA PITZELE

You know what I'm talking about, and we all know that making changes is not easy. To get through the tedium and trauma of chronic illness, we intuitively cling to those routines and habits that we don't have to think about. Unfortunately, because of our illness, those comfortable routines are the very parts of our lives which may have to change the most!

Making changes might be easier if others could *see* our problems. The sight of a wheelchair, a leg in a plaster cast, or a white cane evokes strong and immediate compassion and assistance from most people. But since some of our problems and changes are not always apparent to the casual observer, we don't get much spontaneous support from those around us. We know who we are and what we need, but no one else does. Some of us live in the nether world of the "hidden handicapped."

Changes do not come any easier to us than to anyone else. Slowly, one day at a time, we are all in the process of building and rebuilding a new type of life for ourselves. Every day, we put our credibility and our pride on the line to ask for help and understanding.

I have discovered that changing our concept of what is "normal" is one of the keystones to making the most of our lives. If we can make peace with more conservative, more realistic "new norms," we have a good chance of keeping our self-esteem and a positive self-concept. If we can't make these changes, we are going to lose most of our battles to cope successfully.

Some people call this a lifestyle change; I call it establishing a new normality. We must revise and update our normal standards and expectations for ourselves. If you used to go bike riding, you now may have to be content just to watch. The flight of stairs you used to walk without a second thought has become mountainous, and you may find yourself planning your day just to avoid one more climb. Somehow, you also must learn to explain why you can't finish the errands, make love in the same way, and stay for the whole vacation.

> **"Our desperate chore is to learn to live as well as we can, as soon as we can, in spite of our chronic illness. This means learning from the diagnosis onward not to use pain as a crutch or a shield in our lifes, and learning not to become a chronic complainer or manipulator. Ultimately, we must learn instead to have faith in ourselves and to do the best we can, as often as we can, one day at a time. "**
>
> —SEFRA PITZELE

Our changes affect those around us, too. Our children, for example, who still turn to us as an all-knowing, ever-giving parent, have to adjust to new ways of doing things in the family. This probably means they will have to be more independent, more tolerant, more helpful. Our spouses or friends have to change their expectations, too: Fishing trips and hiking may just not be possible.

Here are some changes you may have to make:

■ Grab more quickly, breathe more deeply, and laugh at yourself for all those times you will "almost" fall.

■ Look people straight in the eye when you talk to them.

- Speak simply, clearly, and without embarrassment when you need help.

- Become selfish by taking better care of yourself so there is something left for everyone else.

- Resist the temptation to exploit your role of "sickie."

- Set new life goals that are meaningful, worthwhile, and achievable.

- Run out of the shadows of guilt and shame, including our own and everyone else's.

- Be proud of what you can do, and not angry or apologetic about what you can't do.

- Stop making excuses for that which you cannot control.

- Regroup (or prioritize) your needs and responsibilities by assigning appropriate priorities to "the important few" instead of "the trivial many."

- Yell only when you get angry, not when you get tired or humiliated.

- Swallow your pride, replace your vanity shoes with sensible footgear, slow down, and begin depending on railings and handholds, especially when crossing marble floors, wet leaves, and icy sidewalks.

- Develop lots of good one-line quips to make good samaritans feel better when they help you pick up your packages. Try something like: "I used to do anti-gravity work for NASA, and sometimes I forget myself."

- Find new friends, and keep old friendships strong.

- Get your telephone directory, workbench, and office desk *really* organized—finally!

- Teach your children that the world will not end if you can't pitch a ball, lift a 20-pound turkey, or tie a fishing lure.

- Listen better.

- Forgive.

- Forget.

- Love more.

Try as we might, none of us will be entirely successful in our efforts to minimize the impact chronic illness has on our lives. Maybe that's okay; maybe we shouldn't try to keep "the big secret" hidden from everyone. Maybe we should call its bluff, dare it to do its worst, and learn to live a rich life in spite of the changes it causes.

" This is a book about redesigning your life, now that you have a chronic illness. It is a book about how to live better, *not just differently*. "

—SEFRA PITZELE

I would like, through this book, to help others move from the time when a chronic disease is overwhelming to the point when the illness finally takes its rightful place as only one facet of an otherwise complete life.

As you read, please think about ideas *you* can share with others with similar conditions. I urge you to contact the local and national associations dedicated to your illness so that others can learn from your experiences. No one has the last word on any illness or condition, including you and me, but we can all help each other help ourselves and those around us.

I have organized the ideas that follow in a sequence approximating the order in which I think you will find them most useful; for example, attitudes, relationships, and feelings are addressed before physical adaptations.

There is an old adage, "Time heals all wounds." I have found that this is not true for those of us who have a chronic illness. The illness stays, even though time passes. But *we* can heal our wounds—if not the physical ones, then at least the emotional wounds caused by long-term illness. By helping each other, we can begin to change. The next steps toward change will have to be yours.

We are *not* alone. Please let me know what you are experiencing. I invite you to contribute to the growing body of knowledge and share what you know with others in similar situations. I want to help you tell others what works and what doesn't. I welcome your suggestions, comments, and questions. You can write me at P.O. Box 16294, St. Paul, Minnesota 55116. (*Every* letter gets answered, but please be patient as I, too, battle with the ups and downs of my illness.)

Most of us remember that our changes began with the first diagnosis. In the next chapter, we'll discuss what the diagnosis really means to you.

FIRST, THERE IS THE DIAGNOSIS

Most of us do not remember precisely when our illnesses began, although many of us suspected we were sick before we were diagnosed by our doctors. Like a faint sound we could not identify, or a shadow just out of sight, an unnamed disease crept into our lives. Like a nagging doubt that could not be chased away, it demanded more and more of our attention.

THE FIRST DIAGNOSIS WAS OUR OWN

Many of us felt vague aches or pains, or ran a fever with some frequency. Others stumbled unexpectedly while walking. Stairs became increasingly difficult to navigate. Some of us had weakened hands, and tried to explain away the broken dishes and dropped tools. "They just slipped and fell," we'd say. Virtually all of us were hesitant to face our physician with such undefined problems. When we finally did, we were usually further confounded by that phrase, "You probably just have some kind of virus."

I call these early feelings *prodromal anxiety*. A prodrome is any symptom which indicates the approach of an illness or condition. Prodromal symptoms such as aches, fevers, and feelings of exhaustion are signals from our body as it tries to warn us of impending problems.

Normally, symptoms are an excellent clue as to what is wrong. Acute illnesses, like the flu or an ear infection, come and go with clear prodromes. Since doctors can diagnose acute problems comparatively quickly and easily, we suffer little anxiety.

Chronic illnesses are different. The prodromes associated with chronic conditions cause much more anxiety because of their perplexing look-alike nature.

In the early stages, many illnesses share prodromes such as exhaustion, weakness, or sore joints. At the time our first prodromes appeared, our symptoms were probably too vague to be clearly linked to an identifiable disease. Nevertheless, we *knew* something was wrong: Too many minor medical problems had occurred, and too much was subtly changing in our bodies. Concern about the unknown kept our doctors and our families guessing.

**"Nothing slows a clock like pain;
Nothing speeds it up like keeping busy. "**

—SEFRA PITZELE

Prodromes also cause anxiety because they are unpredictable. They come and go without warning, pattern, or explanation. Diagnosis is difficult with nonspecific symptoms, placing us in a "well until proven sick" position with our doctors and our families. How can we accurately explain the feeling of total exhaustion that descends upon us unexpectedly while climbing stairs, for example? I know that it's more than just feeling tired: You feel that you cannot go on anymore and that you are at the very bottom of your resources. What can we possibly say to our doctor in the face of such undeniable, yet undefinable, problems?

Perhaps we said nothing at all, and instead convinced ourselves that we were just becoming "klutzy" because we weren't sleeping well or eating right. When we did discuss our symptoms, we ran the risk of boring or annoying our friends and family. They challenged us to prove we weren't hypochondriacs, and perhaps even suspected mental illness.

Naturally, everyone had their favorite home remedy and armchair diagnosis for us, and would quickly lose patience with us when we didn't listen to their advice. Everyone meant well—but of course, just because surgery on his middle ear worked for Uncle Bob when he had similar symptoms does not mean the same treatment will work for us.

To add to the confusion, often our complaints went away entirely, at least for a few months or weeks at a time. This did not help our credibility. How were we to know that these symptoms all pointed to a chronic illness? How were we to know we hadn't just had several cases of the flu?

UNNAMED ILLNESS

I never questioned whether I should believe in myself
Or that I'd not be believed by my doctor and my family.
Because I knew with certainty that I was right.
I never thought I'd lose my credibility just
because I had an unnamed illness.

My
  self
    image
      plummeted as once again I was told:
      "We can find nothing wrong"

Yes
 No
  Yes
   No
    Yes
     No

Perhaps I am not really ill at all.
*How can I believe in **me**,*
If even the doctors aren't sure of what they see?
And so I feel I've lost my credibility.

I don't know where to turn—please help me.

—SEFRA PITZELE, 1982

It is typical to spend months or even years knowing that something is wrong, yet routinely hear that the doctor can't find any problem. We begin to seriously doubt ourselves. We begin to think: Maybe the doctor is right and it was just a flu bug or some new virus. Worse yet, we wonder if maybe we are just getting depressed. We wonder if it is possible that we are just imagining all the aches and pains and disconnected events and signals that seem to be trying to tell us something.

As time goes on, feeling bad—and feeling bad about not feeling well—becomes normal for us, and we forget what it feels like to be healthy. As our confidence in our own judgment erodes still further, we depend more and more on the judgment of those people who seem to have grown numb to our complaints. Before long, we don't know what to believe.

So it goes with the prodromal period, that period of time before a chronic illness is diagnosed. Feeling ill becomes normal, and one loses sight of the old ''norm'' or normal frame of reference. It becomes a vicious merry-go-round: Feel ill, see the doctor, take some tests—and receive no answer. We seem to be stuck in limbo because we can't affirm an illness. We certainly don't *want* to be sick, but the uncertainty is almost as bad as the symptoms. Without a clear diagnosis, we can't even affirm our credibility. A little later, the maddening cycle repeats: Feel ill, see the doctor, leave without a diagnosis, and worry.

It doesn't take very long for us to catch on: The less we say, the less attention we draw to ourselves. We try to ignore our symptoms. Left long enough to run their course, the symptoms eventually become too frequent or too painful or too obvious to ignore.

WHY IS IT HARD FOR YOUR DOCTOR TO MAKE A DIAGNOSIS?

Why can't the doctor make a diagnosis the first time he or she sees us? Many patients resent their physician for what he cannot do, and consequently spend even more money and time seeking different advice, only to be disappointed in the end. This is a trap we must avoid. We need to be realistic about why this continues to happen.

It is one of the paradoxes of chronic illness that we must keep our expectations of our doctor low *before* the diagnosis, and keep them high *after* the diagnosis. Before the diagnosis, your doctor shares your frustration with the unknown and unresolved.

There are several good reasons why your doctor may not be able to give you a definitive answer, and they are rooted in the chronic nature of your illness. We have to face it: Vagueness and uncertainty are part of the nature of every chronic illness or chronic condition. Unlike the acute care problems we are accustomed to, such as broken legs, cuts and viruses, we never are completely "healed" from a chronic illness. Consider that most chronic conditions are caused by:

■ Illnesses that progress slowly, such as multiple sclerosis, rheumatoid arthritis, lupus, or Parkinson's disease.

■ Partial recovery from an acute illness that has some hope for rehabilitation, such as a stroke or encephalitis.

■ Accidents or illnesses that cause permanent and irreversible damage.

The odds of a quick, clear diagnosis—and prognosis (forecast of what is to come)—may be against you and your doctor if your symptoms are caused by one of the circumstances above. Again, the symptoms may just be too vague, or too similar to another illness, for a conclusive diagnosis. As long as the laboratory test results remain within the "normal" range, and the examination reveals nothing unusual, it will be difficult for even the finest diagnostician to name an elusive illness.

This aspect of medicine is frankly as much art as it is science. Mind you, your physician may be relatively certain that a medical problem is beginning, and he may even share that notion with you, but sometimes he will be unable to offer you anything except sympathy. When you return home and report that he found "nothing" again, and nevertheless charged you as if he had, you feel a great need to do *something* to bring this issue to a point of closure.

It is doubtful that your doctor is uncaring or unqualified. He may just be protecting himself—and you—from the consequences of an incorrect diagnosis. He may feel that it is better to wait for clear symptoms and a complete understanding of your condition before embarking on a course of treatment that is possibly long and probably expensive.

He may go so far as to confirm that something *is* wrong with you, but he may be unwilling to speculate what it is because of the physical and financial implications of such a diagnosis. He probably knows better than you what happens when a medical label is assigned to you: It is difficult to get rid of, even if it is later found to be incorrect, and it tends to influence your life dramatically. What if you were given an incorrect diagnosis, and you made significant changes in our lifestyle to accommodate the illness, only to discover later that you had something else entirely?

❝ Happiness should not depend on wellness. ❞

——SEFRA PITZELE

You have two options at this point: Either learn to live with your undiagnosed illness until a distinct, identifiable medical crisis occurs while continuing to see your regular physician, or switch doctors. Neither is a particularly attractive choice.

By this time, most of us are beginning to wonder whether "it's all in our heads." There is certainly nothing imaginary about our frustration, anger, and pain! But clearly, we think, we have to do something; things can't go on like this much longer. What, then, can we do to help speed up the process of the diagnosis?

HELPING YOUR DOCTOR HELP YOU

To make an accurate, early diagnosis, your doctor needs good information about your condition. At this early stage, he will probably be very dependent upon your information because the routine lab tests are likely to be inconclusive. Be aware of how important your description of your symptoms is; it's not enough to drag yourself into the examining room and say, "Something's wrong, Doc. I don't feel so good. Can you tell me what the trouble is?"

First, you have to tell the doctor a lot more than you have before. You have to prepare for a detailed discussion of your symptoms. As soon as the appointment has been scheduled, make yourself sit down and chronicle exactly why you have made this new appointment. Jot down what symptoms you have and when they began. You should also take this time to write out the questions and problems you wish to discuss with the doctor. If this seems time consuming, stick with it anyway. This is *your* problem, and it's worth the extra preparation if you find out what is wrong. Ask yourself:

1. How long have I been feeling ill?
2. What exactly, as I see them, are my symptoms?
3. What has changed from my usual state of health?
4. Have I lost or gained any weight?
5. What do I do that causes pain or discomfort?
6. At what time of the day are the symptoms worst?
7. Have I run a fever? For how long? How high? At what time of the day?
8. Am I getting enough sleep?
9. Have I been under a great deal of stress, either personal or job-related?
10. How have these symptoms changed my daily routine?

Writing down the facts will help you focus on your reasons for going to the doctor for yet another exam, and may help remove some of your self-doubts. And since you're better prepared when you see the doctor, you will get more out of your appointment.

"If I am not for myself, who will be for me?"

—HILLEL

During your appointment, be sure to give your doctor complete and honest information. Don't hide what seems to you to be a minor problem. All the pieces are needed before the doctor can put together the puzzle of your illness. Don't be shy—doctors hear it all. Anything less than complete honesty will only hinder your treatment.

Even after more frank discussions and more tests, you still may know very little. In some cases, your physician may want the professional opinion of one of his colleagues. If he wants a second opinion, he will refer you to a consultant—a physician who has specialized in a particular area of medicine. Generally, your doctor or one of his staff will call the consultant and make the appointment. At the end of this chapter, I have included a list of those types of consultants who would be most likely to treat the illnesses mentioned in this book.

Be patient with your physician, but not for too long. If you are certain you are being misdiagnosed by not being diagnosed at all, it is time to consult with another doctor. Remember, we *own* our bodies, and as the owners, only *we* have read the owner's manual from cover to cover!

THE BEST DIAGNOSIS IS THE LAST DIAGNOSIS

Finally, the day arrives when your symptoms are distinct enough, the right doctor sees the right test data, and you give the doctor enough specific information. For a moment, you can't believe your ears:

"Well, this is interesting. There has been enough of a change for me to make a diagnosis now. You have..."

Finally—a diagnosis! Temporarily, this looks like a gift. No matter what your doctor said, you were probably smiling when you heard the news. At last, the uncertainty is over! You may have still hurt, but you felt relieved. You probably thought to yourself: Good, I *am* really sick, not crazy. There's even a fancy scientific name for what I have, and my friends can look it up in their dictionaries at home and know that I wasn't just imagining all of this.

Other thoughts flood in as the implications of the diagnosis become clear.

"Tell me again what I have," you ask.

"Well, it's a chronic illness," the doctor says, then he spells it for you. Slowly. You try saying it for the first time. Slowly. You fumble for a piece of paper and start writing because you know you won't be able to remember all of this. Then the questions start:

"How will this affect my life? Is it contagious? Is it hereditary? Will I get worse? Do people die from this condition? Am I going to be able to take care of myself? Will I ever get back to normal? How can I handle the medical bills? Will I be able to keep working, or run the house? Am I going to become crippled?"

Your doctor will attempt to answer these preliminary questions. You will think of many, many more. Some you will wish you had never asked. Eventually, one thought crosses your mind: Wait! Doesn't "chronic" mean for the rest of my life? Me, sick forever? A feeling in the pit of your stomach tells you that you are on a roller coaster ride that will make your prodromal worries seem trivial in comparison.

A period of denial is to be expected. As reality crushes in on you, you start looking for a way out. You look for a way to explain your illness away or talk yourself out of it. "Just give me enough time," you think to yourself, "and I'll prove that I am one of those exceptions. My body has always been a little strange anyway. I mean, I'm glad to know finally what I have, but it certainly couldn't be anything *really* serious."

THE DIAGNOSIS

Aha! The wind blows free again!
I was right—and sick I truly am!

Free from the fear of the unknown.
Freed from the fear of not knowing.

Now I have a label—I feel secure once more
*I have a **real** illness—now I know the score.*

I hated the feeling of being in limbo.
But why did I need so badly to know?

For me or for you—or just because I needed the right
to believe in myself again?

——Sefra Pitzele, 1983

Many of us remember being awash with gratitude that our physician finally ventured a concrete diagnosis. But by the time we got home, we could hardly recall what he said. Even worse, we worried because we hadn't really understood what he said, either.

With a diagnosis, we are full of self-affirmation, perhaps even secretly delighted that we are finally believed. Our diagnosis has vindicated us, but it has also presented an entirely new reality. During the days and weeks and months ahead, we will long for blissful ignorance again.

WHAT DOES IT MEAN IF YOU CAN'T GET A DIAGNOSIS?

If you have exhausted your options and still do not have a diagnosis, you have to resign yourself to living with the unknown. It may be some time, perhaps even quite a long time, before you can name what is wrong.

Meanwhile, you are stuck in the twilight zone of the medical arts: You have an undiagnosed chronic condition. You are neither sick nor well. This is precisely the position we are trying to escape with a definitive diagnosis, but it's a fact that some of us will never know any more than we know right now. Our pain, fatigue, and other symptoms are still as real, of course, but they may never be easily explained or predicted.

When a diagnosis is not possible or not forthcoming, you must resolve to make the appropriate changes in your life without it. In spite of your lack of a diagnosis, you can still deal with the symptoms of your condition.

You cannot afford too much time waiting for a diagnosis. The search for a disease is not and should not be the focus of your ongoing doctor-patient relationship. If it is, what will you do after you eliminate all possible diseases?

A diagnosis is a one-time event that provides a useful frame of reference for treatment, nothing more. Most of us have our unique combination of symptoms, anyway. If you and your doctor just acknowledge a set of symptoms, that's enough. Named or unnamed, pain is pain, discomfort is discomfort, and inconvenience is inconvenience.

Regardless of whether or not you have a diagnosis, your focus should still be the management of the chronic medical condition. This management means the maximization of your productivity, creativity, well-being, and happiness. The goals of improving your functioning and satisfaction are usually achieved without curing the underlying disease. Granted, knowing the name of your problem and being able to look it up in the medical books helps a great deal when it comes time to predict the cycles of your condition or when you want to explain what is wrong to your friends and family, but it is not essential. Believe me, your symptoms will continue whether they are named or not, and you have to learn to live with them just the same.

The following three examples will suffice to illustrate the point that the definition of the underlying disease is not always necessary in the management or assessment of chronic illness. Many of us may share these symptoms, yet have quite different treatments. It will make little or no difference if they are ever conclusively linked to a disease.

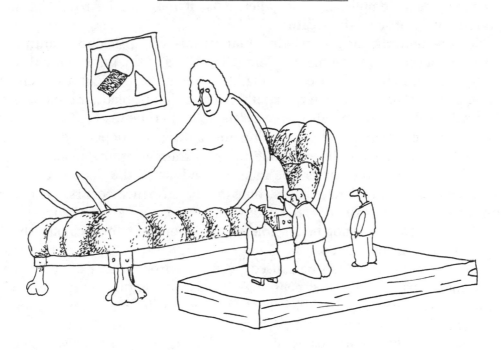

We on the board have decided there's nothing wrong with your head. It's all in your body.

Low-back pain is a symptom in search of a disease. Approximately three-fourths of us will suffer low-back pain with the probability of both remission and recurrence. Low-back pain affects 52 of every 1,000 people in working populations , and 18 of every 1,000 in the same group will be disabled because of it. Despite these high statistics, doctors rarely identify a specific underlying disease. This is a serious problem for many, compromising their ability to dress themselves, to maintain personal hygiene, to move about, and to retain independent functioning.

The management of low-back pain involves education, adaptation of our environment, exercise, and sometimes medication. Further recommendations are tailored to our unique circumstances according to the degree of our incapacitation. Our doctor's advice is directed at the reduction of pain and improvement of our functioning. The identification of the underlying disease may never be accomplished, and when it is, it may not be useful at all in changing or improving the treatment.

Urinary incontinence is the involuntary loss of sufficient quantities of urine to be a social or hygienic problem. Regardless of the underlying disease, urinary incontinence is caused by bladder pressure sufficient to overcome sphincter resistance. It can be the resulting condition of bladder contractions, sphincter weakness, an inability to reach the toilet in time to avoid an accident, or even medications or restraints. Treatment does not depend on knowing whether the bladder instability is due to brain trauma, multiple sclerosis, or other disease. The problem can be managed as long as the doctor knows the mechanism of the problem—that is, how the incontinence occurs. By dealing with the problem successfully, the doctor and the patient avoid the frustration and disappointment of not being able to define or cure the primary disease underlying the incontinence.

Poor hand function can be caused by many chronic diseases such as any one of the arthritic conditions, neurologic disease or complications of diabetes. Many people share diminished levels of function for different reasons, including neurologic or rheumatologic problems.

When your hands are losing strength, does it really matter whether it's from multiple sclerosis or rheumatoid arthritis? The discomfort and inconvenience are the same. Regardless of the reasons, new methods have to be learned to open jar lids, hold a pencil, or use scissors.

This is an example of a chronic condition which is perhaps incurable, but one that can be significantly improved if the focus is on minimizing the discomfort or disability instead of finding the underlying disease. Again, the diseases may be different, but the treatments are similar—to maintain as much hand function as possible. If you are among the sufferers of poor hand function and if you and your doctor are cure-oriented, you both are vulnerable to many disappointments.

SUSAN'S DILEMMA

I have a friend named Susan. For the five years I have known her, I have watched her health go downhill. The other day I watched her, exhausted, trying to function at her counter job and continue to smile and converse with her customers. Later we had a few moments to talk. ''Why,'' I quietly asked her, "are you letting this go on month after month? Does your doctor really know what is going on with you?"

"Because," she told me, "I don't think they believe me anymore. They all see me standing here doing my job, and they have no idea what is really going on with my body. And besides, I know several of them think it's all emotional anyway. It's hard to see so many specialists. No one person really knows what's going on with me. I've been thinking I should see that doctor upstairs. He might help me."

"Sue," I replied, "getting diagnosed is very important, but it's not necessary before you get relief. Your back pain and your hand numbness have to be dealt with right away. Rather than be miserable every day, why not go to that new doctor and let him direct your care. Tell him emphatically that you must have relief, whether you have an illness or not!"

"Okay," she whispered, "I will, I promise. I'll call today."

And she did! To her surprise the doctor listened to her. He said, "Everytime I see you at work you are smiling and talking with the customers. How was I to know you were suffering if you didn't tell me?"

I didn't see Susan for two weeks. When she spotted me she had a grin on her face! "He believed me! He doesn't think I'm nuts! We talked for over an hour. I even told him about some of the smaller problems I'm having. We don't know what's wrong yet, but he wrote me a prescription for physical and occupational therapy, and they are really helping me. He even gave me a muscle relaxant and a prescription for built-up shoes. What a difference in how I feel each day!"

Susan may never be diagnosed, but eventually her symptoms may become serious enough so her disease can be named. It doesn't matter. Now Susan can function with some assurance that there is help available—and that she is credible.

REMAINING UNDIAGNOSED

There are probably as many undiagnosed people in our country as there are those who are diagnosed. So often people write to me and say, "If only this problem had a name, then people would believe in me again, and then I could believe in myself again, too.''

Why should anyone have to suffer for three, ten, or twenty years with the symptoms of a medical problem just because the doctor can't name the illness? Why suffer for more than a few weeks with any symptom before seeking help? Even if you remain undiagnosed you deserve the same excellent medical care as anyone else.

Staying undiagnosed is degrading, frustrating, and often expensive. It can also be very painful, both emotionally and physically. So often the patient sees the doctor, gets no answer, pays another medical bill, and then faces the inevitable questions from friends and family members. "What? You went again and she still doesn't know what's wrong?'' Or, "Why don't you switch doctors? This one must be a quack!'' Silently, they wonder whether the problem is with the doctor's diagnostic technique or your imagination.

If you are one of the thousands who remain undiagnosed, you can still hold your head up high and be proud that you are trying as hard as you can to take care of yourself medically. Continue to believe in yourself. As I said, it *IS* your body and only you have read the owner's manual. In Susan's case, relaxation therapy made all the difference. If you have weak hands, would you rather ask someone to cut your meat for you, or would you rather use a special knife that lets you do the job yourself? I know what my choice was. I carry a special knife in my purse to use when I dine out. Believe me, hardly anyone notices.

Diagnosed or undiagnosed—the problems and pain remain the same. Do the best that you can do for yourself. Be your own advocate. Speak up when you have a special need. You—and how you feel—are very important, whether your medical condition has a name or not. Don't be afraid to look out for yourself.

OTHER SPECIAL PROBLEMS

Everyone's problem is special; the pain and confusion are familiar to all of us. I would like to mention just a few of the other conditions with which people suffer.

Some of the "invisible conditions that don't benefit from high visibility in the media are *endometriosis, chronic yeast infection,* and *PMS, or Pre-Menstrual Syndrome.* It is obvious that these conditions plague women more than men. New treatments and support groups are springing up all over the nation. Women by the scores have written to say, "Hey! We are being forgotten. You only mention the big diseases. We suffer too!'' You are right, of course, and my heart goes out to you.

Another problem which I'd like to mention is that of *orphan diseases*. An orphan disease is one which is very rarely diagnosed, and there are only a few people in any geographical area with the same or similar diseases. There are rarely support groups available for orphan diseases. Legislators have to work incessantly to keep bills going to provide special funds for the development and manufacture of orphan disease medicine. Otherwise, no pharmaceutical house would produce a drug that, say, only two hundred people need. It just would not be cost effective. It is terribly hard to have an orphan disease, but support groups for other illnesses should help you, too. The Epstein-Barr virus is a perfect example.

The problem of *dry eyes*, or *xerophthalmia*, is not at all rare. It can be caused by a disease, such as Sjogren's disease, by a reaction to medicine, aging, or for reasons that are never discovered. If you have never had dry eyes, you have no idea of how disabling it can be. Some people describe it as trying to blink in a sandstorm. Dry eye pain can literally dominate you day and night. Much can and is being done with dry eye treatment and research. It's an uncomfortable and painful condition.

A FEW WORDS ABOUT CANCER

The biggest problem of all is cancer. In previous editions of this book, I carefully avoided listing cancer as a chronic disease because most people still conceive of it as a fatal illness. Believe me when I tell you this is a misconception! I received literally dozens of letters from people who had cancer and were in remission, from those who had active disease, and from their family and friends. They resented being left out, and rightfully so. After all, the family and the patient all suffer the same turmoil, emotions, grief, and pain as any person with any disease.

These folks are playing for keeps in a very high stakes game. The introduction of *Taking Time: Support for People with Cancer* states: ''A diagnosis of cancer . . . is a powerful stimulus against procrastinating on warm and kindly or beautiful things . . . a reminder that many of the material things aren't all that urgent after all. . . . Take time to watch the sunset with someone you love; there may not be another as lovely for the two of you.'' In short, start seeing life with new eyes. There is so much to see.

In some cases cancer is quick and fatal. Take what little time you have to wrap up all the loose ends of your life. Arrange to see your clergyperson. Say ''I love you'' to the people who are most important in your life. And if there is time, arrange for your own funeral. If you can read this book at all, make peace with yourself and all who matter in your life.

By far the largest number of cancer patients have slower-acting disease, or have a period of remission. If you have longer than just a few months, I hope this book can help you and your family. No one with cancer really knows how long they will live. Most hope they will be in the group who achieve permanent or at least long-term remission. You will still have all the same problems and adjustments of others with chronic disease. Occasionally there is a misdiagnosis. Once in a rare while, the cancer stops growing and no one knows why. Keep hoping that a medical breakthrough will occur or that one medical advance will keep you healthy for just a few more years. In the meantime, go about the process of living—not the process of dying.

I'd like to dash the myth that a diagnosis of cancer is always a death sentence. Larger and larger numbers of people who have been diagnosed as having cancer are living long enough to bounce their grandchildren on their knees. Whatever time you have—weeks, months or years—let your diagnosis of cancer remind you of the fragility of life and of relationships.

ACCEPTING THE CHALLENGE OF CHANGE

People respond to their diagnosis in different ways. Some choose not to even talk about their illness with their family or friends. Some go so far as to deny that their doctor said anything at all, choosing to struggle through their daily routines until they are unable to function any longer. Others actually gloat to family and friends that they were right after all, almost punishing those close to them for their votes of no confidence. Of course, there are many more negative than positive ways to handle the diagnosis, and each of us will probably stumble into some of them at one time or another.

If a diagnosis is not possible for your condition, move toward a remedy for your symptoms anyway. You and your doctor cannot afford to spend unlimited time searching and testing for an illness that may not fully emerge for years. A purely disease-specific focus can block you from those treatments that can help you *now*. You and your doctor must begin immediately to think through those strategies that will help you in your larger struggle to adapt to

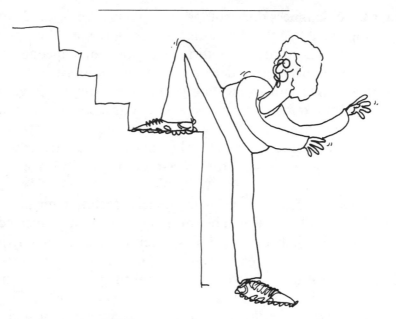

The first step is always the hardest.

new norms. Just because you can't name your problem doesn't mean that you can't help yourself *today*.

Our new challenge is to understand the diagnosis and incorporate what we learn into a new reality for ourselves. Life is going to be different from now on; how we handle the first few weeks after the diagnosis will set the tone for our first big adjustments.

Chronic illness is different from the acute, short-term illnesses like the flu we have known before. Chronic illness is forever. Because our society is oriented toward acute care, we are quite naturally unprepared for the lingering illnesses of others. We are even less prepared for our own.

Now is the time we must take special care of our relationships. We must not allow ourselves, or our loved ones, to overreact. We need support more than ever now, especially from the people we count on to let us sound out our feelings and thoughts without having them make value judgments. In fact, you may find it very helpful to have someone else with you when you meet with your doctor about your illness for the first time. One of you should be free to take notes and give feedback on what the doctor says.

Having a chronic illness does not take away our natural needs for companionship or support. After the diagnosis, our emotions are likely to go into a tailspin, and we will need the unconditional support of someone very close. If we alienate the very person we need most by indulging in self-pity or other counterproductive behavior, we will only end up hurting ourselves in the long run. It is very important to be honest with our feelings, and we need to maintain our relationships in order to get an adult's perspective on our situation. For those of us who already alienated our friends during the prodromal stage of our illness, a little fence-mending and bridge-building may be necessary.

In most cases, it is fair to describe the general feeling after the diagnosis as one of relief. The family is relieved because they have long suspected that there really is a medical problem and now know specifically what they are facing. We are relieved because we are tired of feeling ill and stretching our credibility; we need and are grateful to get medical and family support. Even the doctor is relieved: At last everyone has a specific set of problems to focus on. *The problems have not ended, but they are known and thereby more manageable.*

Most importantly, this experience reminds us that we were indeed listening correctly to the signals our body was sending. That lesson alone is worth many times the cost of our medical care, for we learned to trust our intuitions about ourselves. I like to call this period of time the "honeymoon" period: Everyone is finally focused on specific problems, emotional support is rallied again, and there is a general feeling that no illness or problem is too great to overcome or manage. Frankly, the reality has not set in yet. Welcome to the shortest honeymoon ever! The myths, misconceptions, unrealistic expectations, and immature coping methods are about to be dismantled!

In the few seconds it took my doctor to utter the words, "systemic lupus erythematosus," my life changed forever. So did those of my husband and children. Lupus is an auto-immune disease which causes the body to actually turn against itself and attack tissue such as joints, skin, or even internal organs. The types of changes that occur will differ with the illness, of course. In my case, I was hospitalized; others are placed on medication or started on therapy, and still others may need surgery. In any case, as a treatment program begins, you can count on your doctor to be among your strongest allies. He will doubtlessly be striving to assess the extent and progress of your illness as soon as possible.

BAD NEWS

Bad news.
A lot of it.
All at once.
It feels like a blow.
I stagger, reel.
My eyes blur,
I'm frightened,
And I must confess, God
I feel outraged.
How could you do this to me,
After all I've been through,
Now when I'm already so low . . .
. . . Why me? Why me?
And other men have invented reasons.
All wrong.
There is no reason beyond
My ways are not your ways.
The only thing to do is accept that and go on.
Help me to.
It's hard.
And I'm afraid . . .

——*Excerpted from* Green Winters, A Celebration of Old Age

GETTING ON WITH YOUR LIFE

Even though there are no cures for chronic illnesses, much can be done to improve your quality of life. Just because you are ill does not mean you have to give up your dignity, pleasures, and relationships. Nor does it mean you are excused from contributing your fair share to the rest of the world! It must be your goal to keep yourself as pain-free, productive, and happy as possible.

Now, the challenge is to *manage* your illness and minimize its effects on your lifestyle and livelihood. Because it is difficult to generalize about the effects of chronic illness beyond a certain point, the name of your illness will hardly matter after awhile. What *will* matter is how the illness affects you individually, and what you must do about it as the illness continues to change. Obviously, the illness will continue to dominate your life after the diagnosis until you learn more about it and learn to live with its effects. You will begin by testing your limits, and learning new ways to do old routines.

If you think it's tough for you to learn the truth about your condition, consider what it's like for your family. This adjustment period is a difficult time for everyone. Even though *you* have the disease, your family members suffer right along with you. In our house, we've developed a daily "wait and see" attitude: Each day we wait to see how I'm feeling! In the following chapters, I want to suggest some new ways of dealing with the inevitable changes.

Our education just begins with a diagnosis. Learning what to expect from our illness won't be enough, because our personal worlds are larger than just our bodies. We have to exercise our psychological strengths, expand our options, cultivate attitudes that reinforce us—and then teach what we've learned to those around us!

For example, throughout the adjustment period immediately following the diagnosis, we need to remind ourselves—and our family—that *we* still own our bodies, just as we did before the illness. Our family would like to take control because we are "sick." They are well intentioned, and because they are probably accustomed to dealing only with acute care situations, like the flu or a broken arm, they quite naturally reason that they should or must rush in to take care of us.

Be careful when you begin hearing them say, "You look tired. Go upstairs and rest." They may be right, but you must not let them begin to assume decision-making roles for you. They should be reminded to ask you instead: "You look tired. What can I do to help" They love you, but good intentions will not be enough. There are new sets of rules for everyone. Control is an issue that I will address later in the book; a few simple rules can help make the transition to a new standard of normal much easier.

A diagnosis of chronic illness automatically and unavoidably means that you will always—and I mean *always*—have an illness in your home. Some of us will be lucky enough to go into remission, which means that no symptoms are evident and no medicines are required. Others will be able to achieve suppression, which means that no symptoms are evident with the aid of medicine. Others will progress in the slow but unrelenting pattern of their illness. Unfortunately, many of the more slowly progressing diseases have been at work in our bodies for years prior to the diagnosis, making them difficult to control.

Nevertheless, when we get to it, the diagnosis offers us a freedom we have probably not had for some time: We finally know what we are fighting. Once the uncertainty of an undiagnosed condition is removed, we can manage our lives accordingly. At least with a name for our condition and a basic understanding of what is going to happen to our bodies, we can make plans again and get on with our lives, even if those plans must include chronic illness.

The diagnosis is actually the beginning of a new kind of life for you. It is a benchmark, a new chapter, a different road to travel. It is not the end of your "healthy" life, but rather the end of not knowing what is wrong.

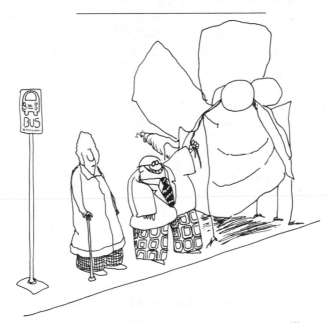

Abner is glad he just has a bug instead of a chronic illness.

CONSULTANT GLOSSARY

Anesthesiology: The branch of medicine which studies anesthesia and anesthetics. An **Anesthetic** is a drug or agent used to abolish sensation of pain, or an agent which blocks nerve conduction or can be applied directly to the area to be anesthetized.

Cardiologist: A physician of internal medicine who has taken further study in the treatment of heart disease.

Chiropractic: A system that teaches that all illnesses are caused by pressure on the spinal nerves, and can be corrected by adjustment to the spine.

Chiropractor: A person who uses the methods taught as chiropractic. A chiropractor is not a medical doctor.

Dermatologist: A physician who has specialized in disorders of the skin.

Endocrinologist: A physician who has completed further medical training in endocrinology, the diagnosis and treatment of disorders in the glands of internal secretion, i.e., the endocrine glands.

Family Practitioner: A medical doctor who has had further training in family medicine, and who has been trained to take care of the whole family, from pregnancy through geriatrics.

Gastroenterology: The study of the stomach and the intestines and their diseases.

General Practitioner: A medical doctor who treats the whole family, from pregnancy to geriatrics, but who has not had further training in the care of families.

Geriatrician: A specialist in the treatment of the aged.

Hematologist: A specialist in the study of the blood and blood-forming tissues.

Infectious Disease Specialist: A specialist who studies and treats infectious disease.

Intern: A graduate of a medical (or dental) school serving in a hospital preparatory to being licensed to practice medicine or dentistry. An intern is *not* a doctor of internal medicine.

Internist: A physician who specializes in the diagnosis and medical treatment of diseases of adults. An internist does not focus on surgical or obstetrical treatment.

Nephrologist: A physician of internal medicine who has been further trained to study the science, function, and disease of the kidneys.

Neurologist: An expert in neurology, which is the treatment of disorders of the nervous system.

Neurosurgeon: A physician who has further specialized in both neurology and surgery and performs surgery on the nerves.

Obstetrician: One who practices the branch of medicine and surgery that deals with the management of pregnancy, labor, and the puerperium.

Occupational Therapy: The branch of therapy that teaches or re-teaches activities needed for daily living skills or for work.

Ophthalmologist: A physician who has further specialized in disorders of the eye and who performs eye surgery.

Optometrist: A *dispensing* optometrist helps fit glasses and can perform a visual check-up. He is not a physician. A *fitting* optometrist takes the order for the glasses and grinds it according to the prescription. He is not a physician.

Orthopedist: A physician who deals with correction or prevention of disorders involving the bones, joints, muscles, tendons, and ligaments. Orthopedists perform surgery as well.

Osteopathy: A school of medicine based upon the theory that a normal body, when environment and nourishment are satisfactory, can work to re-establish its health. Using manipulative, physical, and surgical methods, the osteopath works to restore function and internal balance to the patient.

Otolaryngologist: A physician who specializes in the medical and surgical treatment of the head and neck, including the ears, nose, and throat.

Pediatrician: A physician who specializes in that branch of medicine which treats the child and his or her development, and diagnoses and treats the diseases of children.

Pharmacist: One licensed to prepare and dispense drugs.

Physiatrist: A physician with further training in rehabilitative medicine.

Physical Therapist: A person trained to help patients regain endurance, muscle tone, and perhaps prevent some deformities.

Psychiatrist: A physician with further training in psychiatry, the branch of medicine that deals with the study, treatment, and prevention of mental illness.

Psychologist: A specialist in psychology, the branch of science that deals with the mind and mental processes, especially in relation to human and animal behavior.

Pulmonologist: A medical doctor concerned with the anatomy, physiology, pathology, and diseases of the lungs.

Radiology: That branch of medicine concerned with radioactive substances, including X-rays and the application of information to help prevent, treat, and diagnose disease.

Rheumatology: The branch of medicine dealing with rheumatic disorders, their causes, pathology, diagnosis, and treatment.

Social Worker: A specialist who works with the patient or his family to solve their problems, often in this context related to illness, medical care, financial, or physical care problems.

Speech Pathologist: A person trained in the pathology of speech who works with speech or memory problems to help the impaired person gain or re-gain optimum use of speech and memory.

Urologist: A physician who practices the branch of medicine concerned with the urinary tract in both sexes and the genital tract in the male.

—*Source: Adapted primarily from* **Dorland's Illustrated Medical Dictionary,** *Twenty-sixth Edition, Philadelphia, et al., 1974.*

GRIEVING IS NORMAL

*I*t's true, friends—you appreciate most that which you have lost.

I remember such a moment shortly after my first conclusive diagnosis. I was in my hospital bed, someone had just left me after a visit, and I found myself staring at the afternoon sunlight on the far wall. Suddenly, the hospital became very quiet, and time seemed to stand still. A terrible feeling crept into me, and I began to cry. It sounds crazy, but I felt as if I'd lost something very dear to me. I didn't know what it was, but I knew it was gone forever.

Later, I learned that my acute sense of loss was a signal that I was unconsciously beginning to understand my illness and what it would mean to me. I wish someone had told me at the time that this was normal, predictable, and something I needed. As it was, I struggled too long to put a brave face on everything and I spent too much time pretending for the sake of others.

In the post-diagnosis euphoria, you were perhaps temporarily relieved, even elated, to end the uncertainty of your condition. You didn't yet understand the full implications of your diagnosis. But a day, a week, perhaps a month later, the honeymoon period with your chronic illness comes to an end once and for all. Your attention will soon shift from the disease you have acquired to all that you have lost.

The process by which we acknowledge and come to terms with our losses is known as grieving. Although grieving is usually associated with death, it follows *any* kind of a loss, including the loss of a job, the loss of valuable personal possessions, or in our case, the loss of control over our bodies and our lost opportunities. While you are going through a period of grief, you may be so overwhelmed that you wonder if you will ever recover. Nonetheless, grief follows a consistent pattern that eventually leads to a resolution.

It is an article of faith in mental health circles that grieving must occur before a person can accept a loss. It is the way our emotions "let go" of what once was in order to make room for the changes that will be. When we deny our feelings and the grieving process, we postpone the inevitable maturation of our emotions and hinder our progress toward a happier, more realistic future.

After talking with many other sufferers of chronic conditions and professional counselors, I have a few observations that you may find interesting in light of your situation.

WHY ARE WE GRIEVING?

We grieve for ourselves. We are sad because of what we have lost, including our health, our normal routines, and the future opportunities that will never be. I grieved for the loss of control of my body, my sense of well-being, and all those things which I might no longer be able to do.

I think we all grieve for something else, too: The death of our idyllic images of ourselves. I discovered myself wanting to play tennis and go on a long bike ride soon after I began feeling my acute sense of loss. Never mind that I rarely played tennis before and avoided bike riding by letting the air out of my tires! I sadly had to confront reality and revise my self image. All of my dreams, interpretations, and foolishness were going to have to change.

Some of us try to deny this fundamental, inescapable fact by grimly soldiering on with our "normal" lives. For a while we may even manage to maintain the illusion. Eventually, however, our illness catches up with us, and our dreams become casualties of our illness. For example: A 39-year-old woman on her way up the corporate ladder is forced to change jobs because multiple sclerosis has diminished her ability to speak clearly. As a result of his lung disease, the athlete who had hoped to compete in the Boston Marathon now finds himself puffing after walking the dog around the block. The housewife who had hoped to attend evening classes and finally earn her degree can now barely open a book or hold a pencil because of joint inflammation from rheumatoid arthritis. While chronic illness isn't usually fatal in the physical sense, we do experience the death of our old images of who we are and what we are able to accomplish.

But unlike physical death, we have the capacity to come back from the psychological deaths we suffer as a result of our illness. The first step is to "bury" most of our old selves and our old goals. Only by recognizing that most of our dreams and hopes can never be fulfilled as we planned can we begin the long, slow process of building a new life. If we struggle to hang on to what we've lost, we will only ruin the opportunities that remain for us.

❝To suffer is not the worst thing that can happen to us; the worst thing is not to believe in anything worth suffering for.❞

——SARAH PATTON BOYLE

OUR FAMILY GRIEVES, TOO

As much as my grieving was a surprise to me, my family's grieving was a real eye-opener. Looking back, what happened makes sense, but it was traumatic at the time. My husband had to say good-bye forever to part of our life together. Perhaps he was disappointed in more ways than I was. Perhaps he was carrying dreams and interpretations and foolishness, too.

He told me at the time that the most frustrating aspect of my illness was that he could not control what was happening. Eventually, we learned that we both had more control over our lives than we first thought, but we felt powerless for a long time after the diagnosis. There did not seem to be anything we could do to help ourselves or stop a bad situation from developing. The more we talked, the more I came to understand that he had a very rich and complex picture of me as wife, lover, mother of his children, soulmate, partner, and friend. My illness was causing him to dismantle many of those pictures, one by one, against his will. He was grieving, too.

My children were sad, too. They were also fearful. All they understood for certain was that their mother was sick a lot more, and that they could not see me as much, and that all the adults they knew were very worried about something terrible. More than once, their imaginations and fears got the best of them. Was Mom going to die? Was Mom ever going to be able to play again? Why didn't she cook anymore? Didn't Mom care about how they did in school anymore? In their way, they also were saying good-bye to what they knew and preparing for change.

UNDERSTANDING THE GRIEVING PROCESS MAKES IT EASIER

Neither my husband nor I realized at the time that we were grieving. We spent a lot of time "sparring" with each other just because we were frustrated, worried, pretending, resentful, and fearful. Of course, I could only see things from my viewpoint. After all, *I* was the one who was so sick. *I* was the one in pain. *I* was the one who had to make the major adjustments. For a while, I could not see that those around me were also hurting. I wasn't even willing to acknowledge that my husband *had* a viewpoint. "Why," I thought at the time, "can't he just shut up and help me deal with this?"

Looking back on those terrible months, I wonder how any of us made it. Each of us was moving through the phases of grief at our own pace, and we all seemed to be in different stages at different times. You can imagine the complicated emotional havoc a family goes through. It was chaos for us! Here we were, a family that seemed to have so much going for us, pushing each other away instead of pulling together! If this was what the rest of my life looked like, I wanted no part of it!

All of us were hurting. Illness does not affect one member of a family without causing a "ripple effect" that touches other family members and friends. My illness was causing problems for everyone. My husband was trying to cope with my roller coaster feelings, the children's fears, his own worry, and at the same time put dinner on the table and finish the laundry. He could see that because I was changing, he was going to have to change, and he didn't know how to deal with that.

No one explained to us that our feelings of loss and pain were normal. Not only were we *supposed* to hurt, but acknowledging our losses should have been one of the healthiest activities we could have done for ourselves and for each other. It would have helped so much if we had been able to share *all* of our feelings with each other.

THE FIVE PHASES OF GRIEVING

Clinically speaking, there are fives stages of grief which we must pass through following a loss. These are:

1. Denial and Isolation.
2. Anger.

3. Bargaining.
4. Depression.
5. Acceptance.

Let's look at each of these stages and try to understand them a little better so that we can appreciate what is happening to us. Perhaps if we are better prepared for the strong feelings that are headed our way, we can get our loved ones and ourselves out of the way before permanent damage is done!

Stage 1, Denial and Isolation: The first stage of the grieving process is a defense mechanism. Denial usually lasts only for a short time. It allows us to collect our thoughts. What is really happening to us? What have we been told? We need some time to adjust intellectually to what our doctor has said to us. We need some time to wonder if the doctor is correct, too.

Denial is the mental numbness that follows a severe emotional wound. For a brief period, we might not feel *anything*. Because we are not quite ready to grasp the full implications of what has happened, we dismiss it, rationalize it, or question its truth:

> "So I slur my words a little bit. No one's *really* going to notice. Surely they'll be more interested in *what* I'm saying rather than the *way* I say it."

> "Doctors have been wrong before. I *know* I can still run marathons. I just have to rest more and take extra vitamins."

> "A chronic illness! But it *can't* be! I've just registered and paid my tuition for law school!"

Denial is normal. It is one of the first defense mechanisms of our conscious mind. You have experienced it at other times in your life, too. Remember when your first pet died? You may have told yourself it was "just resting" until you were ready to acknowledge the truth. Denial gives us time to catch our emotional breath.

Dr. Shlomo Breznitz, an Israeli psychologist, has identified seven levels of denial a person uses to relieve anxiety, including the stress caused by a loss. The less threatening the event, the lower the level of denial.

Level I: Denial of Personal Relevance: "So what! I have a chronic illness. Big deal. I can handle it."

Level 2: Denial of Urgency: "I've got plenty of time. It takes years to develop."

Level 3: Denial of Vulnerability: "I know someone with the same thing, and you can hardly tell."

Level 4: Denial of Feelings: "I don't care if it slows me down some, I'll just do other things."

Level 5: Denial of Source of Feelings: "I've been a little tired lately, but it's not because of my illness."

Level 6: Denial of Threatening Information: "Now they are saying it can cause brain problems. Ridiculous. Don't bother me about it."

Level 7: Denial of All Information: "What a bunch of loonies you guys are. If you want to believe that it causes kidney disease, go ahead. I don't believe a bit of it."

For different life events, we use different levels of denial. This is perfectly normal. It gives us time to deal either with the problem (or the fear), or to move to a higher level of denial.

Some people try to deny their illness in actions as well. The young woman executive may continue to make presentations in spite of her increasingly severe speech problems; the runner might undertake a regimen of resting and exercising, trying to maintain his breathing ability; the aspiring homemaker/ law student might determinedly begin to attend classes, in spite of her rheumatoid arthritis. Denial never lasts long, however. Sooner or later, the limitations imposed by our illness can no longer be ignored. Then, the anger sets in.

Stage 2, Anger: Anger is a terrifying and ugly emotion that most of us would prefer to avoid. Most of us have been brought up to think of anger as impolite, childish, or sinful. As a result, we usually feel guilty when we display angry behavior. Nevertheless, we shout at our loved ones for no reason and brood about the injustice of God, life, and the universe.

If we are ever to work our way through grief, we must learn to set aside our old taboos about anger and accept it for what it is: A normal and even a necessary emotion. Recognizing and expressing anger is painful, but the consequences of ignoring it are far worse. As Dr. Theodore Rubin points out in his excellent and useful *Angry Book*, repressed anger manages to appear in a wide variety of ugly disguises, including sarcasm, gossip, compulsiveness, and prejudice. Suppressed anger can also cause headaches, backaches, stomach problems, and other ailments. Those of us with chronic illness cannot afford to make matters worse for ourselves either mentally or physically.

Anger often takes the form of an intense feeling of unfairness. For example, the young executive might ask, "Why did this have to happen to *me*? I could have done so much for the company if it hadn't been for this stupid disease!" When we are angry, minor frustration can often trigger inappropriate outbursts.

At one time, the aspiring marathon runner might have prided himself on his ability to remain cool under pressure. He now finds himself pounding the walls of his office when he cannot catch his breath. Anger becomes most problematic when it starts affecting innocent bystanders like our family and friends. The student/homemaker might have been a fairly calm, easy-going parent before her illness. But since the onset of her disease, she finds herself launching into a tirade when her children ask a simple question like, "When will dinner be ready, Mom?"

Without question, the anger phase is one of the most difficult to live through. And there are no miracle solutions. We can only ride it out as best we can. Gradually, and with effort, we can learn appropriate ways to express our anger, but it will never disappear completely. For example, instead of lashing out at our nearest and dearest, we might instead retire to a private place to pound pillows, kick tires, or scream. On those unavoidable occasions when we *do* lose control, we may learn to explain to those we affect that we aren't angry at *them*. You must tell them that, on the contrary, you could not cope with your illness at all without their love and support. We are angry at our *condition*, and we will need some time to learn to adjust to it. For particularly tough episodes, psychological counseling can be invaluable to understand the reasons for our anger and to learn better ways to express it. Let me emphasize again that anger is a part of our emotional make-up and a part of the grieving process. We cannot avoid it without risking harm to ourselves and others, but we can learn to handle it.

Stage 3, Bargaining: The third stage in the model, bargaining, may occur simultaneously with any of the others. It rarely lasts very long, simply because we soon recognize its futility. In this stage, we try to cure ourselves with good intentions:

"If I'm allowed to race, I won't sell out like other big name athletes. I promise I won't turn into a huckster for running shoes or deodorant or breakfast food.''

"If I make it through law school, I'll dedicate my life to fighting child abuse.''

"If only I can get in remission, I promise I'll never get angry at the kids again.

"Oh, please, let me get better. This is the only job I could get and I gotta feed my wife and kids.''

Unfortunately, no matter how good we have been, are, or intend to be, bad things like chronic illness can still happen to us. Trying to account for this fact of life and trying to bargain it away are both exercises in futility.

Stage 4, Depression: Depression sets in with the realization that neither rage nor good intentions will make our disease go away. It is through depression that we recognize that the deepest emotion that our illness has caused is sadness. This stage is by far the longest, and one that can recur frequently. Sometimes, just when we seem to be coming to terms with our illness, depression rears its ugly head again. We must not let the unpredictability of depression throw us into despair. Again, it is a predictable phase in the normal process of grieving.

In a sense, denial, anger, and bargaining are attempts to avoid confronting our intense pain at the loss of our health, hopes, and dreams. With the onset of depression, we are cornered at last by our pain. We can only free ourselves by *feeling* it, fully and honestly. Because these feelings are so powerful and so deeply rooted, we must allow ourselves enough time to resolve them.

"Never allow your own sorrow to absorb you, but seek out another to console, and you will find consolation. "

—J.C. MAUCAULAY

With depression, you can expect unpredictable tears. You may start to cry at the most unexpected times and for the smallest reasons. The business-woman with multiple sclerosis might break down while watching a simple story on TV. The sight of the local courthouse might reduce the law student/ arthritis victim to tears. The superficial causes of their tears might appear trivial, even absurd, but they are all-too-vivid reminders of the losses in their lives. Don't push away your need to cry.

Of course, not everyone going though depression bursts into tears. Some people sob silently; that is, they experience intense sadness, but do not express it in obvious tears. Whether sadness takes the form of noisy sobbing or frozen misery, we must allow it to run its course.

Depression can become so severe that basic, day-to-day functioning be-comes impossible. Signs of dysfunction that might indicate a major or severe depression requiring professional intervention include:

- Feelings of sadness which last "far too long" in relation to the event.

- Drastic changes in sleeping patterns, such as sleeping too much or hardly at all.

- Listlessness.

- A decreased ability to concentrate.

- Extreme feelings of guilt.

- Thoughts of, or attempts to commit suicide.

- Eating too much or too little.

- A sense of worthlessness.

- Sexual dysfunction.

If your feelings of sadness reach a point where you can no longer cope with them, get help! The normal feelings of depression attached to grief can and must be worked through, but it is almost impossible to cope with severe depression without professional help. For a more thorough discussion on depression, please see Comments on Depresseion, pages 143-150.

In the depressed phase of our grieving, we may feel that our useful and worthwhile lives are over. If we can't be a company president, an athlete, a lawyer, or achieve any of our other vanished dreams, we may wonder what we have left to live for. As time passes and depression diminishes, we regain a sense of proportion. You will realize that although your illness has closed some of life's paths, the journey can proceed on other, equally challenging and exciting routes.

Begin taking stock of what remains, rather than fixating on what is lost. Try to learn more about your illness so you are better able to cope with your symptoms and limitations. Once you acquire a more balanced sense of what you can and can't do, you can begin to set new goals for yourself. This reassessing and rebuilding characterizes the final stage of grieving, acceptance.

Stage 5, Acceptance: Let's look at how our three hypothetical chronic illness victims arrive at the stage of acceptance. The young executive with multiple sclerosis, for example, discovers an equally challenging position elsewhere in her company. The would-be marathon runner finds that coaching winners is as rewarding as being one. The aspiring law student learns that the legal profession is not entirely closed to her. She may not have the energy or strength to handle three grueling years of law school, but she can manage several months of paralegal training at the local community college. And as a paralegal, she has much more flexibility with her working hours.

In the process of acceptance, we actually discover sometimes that our old goals may not have been possible or feasible even if we had remained healthy. If nothing else, chronic illness instills a certain sense of realism.

It's important to note that understanding the five stages of grieving does not allow you to control, avoid, or cheat the process. Understanding helps only because it makes it a bit easier. You recognize that you are going through a normal adjustment and that, given time, the hurt will pass.

Sidney Greenberg, in *A Treasury of Comfort,* suggests the following ways to help someone in sorrow:

1. Don't try to "buck them up."
2. Don't try to divert them.
3. Don't be afraid to talk about the person who has passed away.
4. Don't be afraid of causing tears.
5. Let them talk.
6. Reassure—don't argue.
7. Communicate—don't isolate.
8. Perform some concrete act.
9. Swing into action.
10. Get them out of themselves.

Chronic illness does eliminate many of our choices in life and, quite understandably, we grieve for our lost opportunities. Nevertheless, some choices do remain for us, no matter how disabled we are. No matter how many dreams we have lost, we can choose to appreciate what remains and set new goals, rather than despair over our losses. We can use our remaining abilities to make a contribution, rather than dwell on our misfortunes. We must do what can be done, rather than brood futilely over what can't be done. We can use our illness as a means to find a richer and more fulfilling life. The decision is ours.

CIRCLE OF TIME

Does the time of grieving ever end?
Or does it just keep rotating like the earth around the sun or the hands around the clock?

Will I ever be free of the anger I feel when I look in the mirror?
I know that underneath all this cortisone fat is the "real me"—but I have lost sight of who I used to be.

*I need to learn that I am what I am **now**—and so I still grieve.*
It comes in spurts, more often in the evening, when I am tired or alone with my private thoughts.

I think the old me will never really come back again.

Time is one thing I have far too much of now.
And I am tired of waiting.

——*SEFRA PITZELE, 1984*

IN SICKNESS AND IN HEALTH...

Explaining your illness to those you love

Y ou won't be able to hide your chronic illness from your loved ones. They have a front row seat at a home movie they never wanted to see. You are the reluctant center of attention, watching them watch you.

You can't keep your illness from affecting them. In many ways, they are going to hurt just as much as you, perhaps more. Your doctor will probably not tell you about this side effect common to all chronic illnesses: The heart ache.

"Not me," we all say, shortly after the diagnosis. "*My* husband (or wife or friend or sibling or parent) is different. Love conquers all. Our love for each other has gotten us through plenty of tough times before, and it will get us through this, too."

Good for you, for now. That idealism will support you both for awhile. But I want to caution you against trusting too much in blind faith. Instead, I urge you to change your relationships, especially your communication patterns, early enough in your illness to help you keep your relationship together. Because chronic illness is forever, you won't be able to "get through" it the way you would an acute illness, a broken leg, or other problem with a distinct beginning and end.

Chronic illness tends to smash people together, and then it drives them apart. Chronic illnesses can control relationships, make them fragile, and rip them like a tissue when we forget to be careful. In this chapter, I would like to make you aware of the symptoms that suggest your illness is unnecessarily hurting your most important relationships. I would also like to share a few practical ways of dealing with these problems.

FOREWARNED IS FOREARMED

The case for close, loving relationships that function well probably does not have to be argued here. You already intuitively know the value of these nurturing relationships. They give us a reason to get up every day, a purpose, a sense of esteem and dignity, and much, much more. Mentally, emotionally, spiritually—they are our sustenance. Take them away, and we are colder, lonelier, and less than our best.

The relationships I want to focus on here are the ones that are the most important to us. I want you to think about the one or two people in your life who are central to your happiness. This "central person" might be your husband or wife, a sister or brother, or a long-time friend. It's the person with whom you can share and relate in a very close and caring way on a regular basis. You may not live with this person or share an intimate physical relationship, but he or she is at least someone you speak with or see frequently. Your children don't qualify for this type of peer relationship, although you may be close to them (we'll address those relationships in the next chapter). For discussion, let's presume the central person is your spouse.

TO MY HUSBAND

When the Rabbi said to us that winter day in '63
"Will you love and care for him or her no matter what you see?"
We never knew the future held for us a long-term ill
Something time won't rectify and won't pass with just a pill.

An illness which has caused us both to search our very beings.
Can we truly stay together when at forty
We should just be freeing
Ourselves of the bonds of children so young—
Just when our real adult lives together should have begun?

Do you love me enough to stand by my side?
Is there goodness enough to keep me your bride?
For I intend to keep living, keep loving, keep hoping
Since being alone only leads to moping.

I have seen us grow so much these past few years
And time and love seem to lay to rest the deepest of our fears.

Through the sadness, through our clinging
Came the laughter and the tears.

And soon we realized that inside I am still just me—
Struggling with illness to achieve autonomy.

I am growing day by day
And we have made decisions, and we will try to stay—together.

For nothing lasts forever and soon things will improve
And I'll still be your helpmate and you'll be my handsome groom.

We've surely changed and grown as my illness took its toll,
But slowly, oh so slowly, we've each learned our brand new role.

Yes, I'd stay with you in illness and through changes till the end,
For I love you, I'm committed, and I want you for my friend.

True love should stand the real-life test of pain, of change, of time.
We've learned so much since we were young, and we are doing fine.

——SEFRA PITZELE, 1982

It is helpful to acknowledge that steering a marriage through any crisis is risky business. It's easy to stay together when the relationship looks like the best place to be, right? In these circumstances, a crisis can actually pull a family together for awhile. Short-term difficulties can cause them to set aside their personal agendas and rise above personal problems in order to help one another.

The story is different when the crisis stops being a crisis and starts being a chronic condition. People are people, not heroic cartoon characters who commit their lives to hopeless quests, thankless tasks, and noble gestures just because "it's the right thing to do." We live in the real world, where real people get tired of fighting, sometimes give up, and always change.

We must remember that chronic illness does not affect us alone. Our loved ones often have to sit by and watch us decline, physically, mentally, or spiritually, because of our condition. They may not share our physical symptoms, but they too suffer fear, anger, and grief. They also are forced to come to terms with the impact the illness has made in their life plans and roles.

**"For every achievement there is a price.
For every goal there is an opponent.
For every victory there is a problem.
For every triumph there is a sacrifice."**

—WILLIAM ARTHUR WARD

In our world, change and illness cause stress, and stress contributes to the breakdown of relationships. When a profoundly handicapped child is born, the statistical odds of his or her parents staying together drops by 50 percent. The divorce rate is almost as high when the crisis involves a partner who suddenly experiences a radically different medical condition. The slower the progression of the illness, the better the opportunity to change the relationship. Close to 75 percent of all marriages in which one partner has a chronic medical condition fail.

With enough time and enough communication, people *can* incorporate into their relationships the new norms and expectations brought on by chronic illness. If you have a relationship you want to keep, start the healing and building process now. Today. I will be the first to agree that having the benefit of someone else's hindsight may not give you all the insight you need to save a marriage, but it may help you just enough to begin the process of change a little sooner. For some, this can make all the difference.

RELATIONSHIPS THAT FUNCTION WELL DON'T JUST HAPPEN

Our best relationships are those that function well. We may not know precisely why, but in most circumstances, they work. The lines of communication are generally clear of static, misunderstanding, confusion, and distrust. In smooth-functioning relationships we solve problems efficiently, share openly, and foster positive, supportive feelings for each other.

Notwithstanding the marriages that are made in heaven, these relationships work because we care enough to work at making them the best they can be. It isn't easy. They require significant investments of time and effort, and above all, they require the practice of certain skills.

Here's what you have to keep in mind: If you and your spouse are going to successfully accommodate chronic illness in your relationship, some things will have to change. Just as you will have new definitions for "normal" in other areas of your life, your central relationship will require new and better skills.

If you let it, your chronic illness will change the orientation of your relationship away from nurturing each other and towards nurturing *it*. Your illness can become the focus of your relationship, making an awkward triangle: You, your spouse, and *it*.

Think about your home. How well do you think you and your spouse are communicating about your illness? Do these sound familiar yet?

"I know I said I would clean out the garage today, but my legs were bad. I just didn't get to it. I promise I'll try tomorrow."

"Why do you kids always start to pick at one another when I'm tired?"

"John, I'm tired, too. I have to put up with your illness, so you'll just have to put up with my crabbiness."

"I'm sick of trying to be heroic. I'm no damn angel of mercy."

"Dr. Thompson says I had better get a walker. He told me that I might fall because my legs are getting so weak. I'm scared, honey. And I'm ashamed because you're embarrassed for me."

"What do you mean we can't go? You promised me, didn't you? Your stupid illness gets in the way of everything."

"I wish I'd never heard of muscular dystrophy. It's ruined all of our plans for the future."

"Why do I always feel so guilty that so much of our money is being spent for my medical bills? If it were you or one of the children, I wouldn't feel so bad."

"I hate this damn illness. Everything I ever planned for myself is ruined. Why don't you go out and have some fun? There's no reason both of us have to sit on the sidelines."

"Sure, it's true: If I'd never been sick, I wouldn't have met all these terrific people. But you know what? I wouldn't have missed them. There are terrific people out in the healthy world, too, and I could have met them just as easily."

"If my husband were still alive, he would help me with the chores I never seem to get done. I sure miss him."

"Why do you keep asking me to do things you know I can't do? Sometimes I think you do that just to be mean to me."

"Stop crying, you big baby. All you ever do is complain."

"Look, I'm sorry. I thought you would be too tired to go. It was an honest mistake. You know I try to include you."

"I see you broke another dish today. Maybe we should invest in a company that makes paper plates so we can pay some of these bills."

"Do you know how angry I am that I don't even have the strength to pick up my grandson? I wish that Dr. Silver had never told me about the multiple sclerosis. What I didn't know wasn't going to hurt me."

"I don't want to talk about it. I'm fine, just fine."

No matter what words I put on paper about the reality of chronic illness, they all seem mild compared to what really happens in your home and mine.

There is hope, though. We do *not* have to give up our most important relationships just because we're sick, and we do *not* have to watch them fall apart or drift apart just because they weren't perfect to begin with.

The most important skills that you and your partner have to improve are your communication skills. If you haven't had your first major-league misunderstanding yet, you may not believe me, but you will soon learn that you need a new vocabulary and a new set of interpersonal "signals" to communicate about your illness. We no longer have the old options of stomping out of the room, arguing vehemently for long periods, distracting ourselves by "getting away," or retreating to our jobs.

As long as we realize we can and must improve the functioning of our communication patterns within our relationships, there is hope. The following pages cover some of the most important issues that will confront you.

“Faults are thick where love is thin. ”

—DANISH PROVERB

CHRONIC ILLNESS WILL NOT CORRECT OR HIDE THE PROBLEMS IN YOUR RELATIONSHIP

Your illness may bring out some of the best aspects of your personality, such as determination and patience, but it will also bring out some of the worst. It has the same effect on relationships. The problems you and your partner were having before the diagnosis will persist until you correct them. If the two of you had a difficult time making decisions about priorities, or talking about money, or relating to each other physically, you are probably still going to have to keep working to improve those aspects of your relationship.

Just like other people, sick or not sick, your problems do not go away by themselves. It is tempting to throw up your hands and say, "I'm not well. How can I deal with *that*?" or "I don't think that's important anymore. Why don't we talk about real problems—like mine?" It's not fair to use the illness as an excuse to quit on your partner, or yourself, or your relationship. You still have a responsibility to care and share and participate in your relationship like an adult.

Your perspective may change, however. Your illness, or the illness of your partner, may change the way you think about your problems and the way you approach them. You both may decide that some of the old issues are not issues any longer. Or, you both may decide that your time together is too precious to spend it discussing trivial differences. If a chronic illness has one beneficial effect, it is to hasten the process of change. These changes can be very positive if you know what you are trying to improve.

WHY

Why a tragedy?
Why not a reason for new experiences?
Why a tragedy?
Why not a way to reach out to people?
Why a tragedy?
Why not the first day of the rest of your life?
Life can be a triumph or a tragedy.
So can chronic illness.
Why must it always be a tragedy?
Triumph for a change!

——*Sefra Pitzele, 1986*

YOU EVENTUALLY MUST TELL YOUR PARTNER THE WHOLE TRUTH ABOUT YOUR ILLNESS

The important people in your life have a right to an accurate picture of the situation. Like you, it is hard for them to adjust, and they will be better prepared if they know all the facts.

Some of us do not tell ourselves the truth about our condition, and that makes telling someone else practically impossible. You won't be able to say what needs to be said until you have come to terms with it yourself.

You can imagine the kinds of information you would want if the situation were reversed. You would want to hear:

"Honey, I'm sick. And I'm not ever going to be completely well again. But I *will* get better."

"I love you."

"I still need you."

"I still need to know you need me."

I have found an incredible amount of strength and courage and satisfaction in simple, straightforward conversations. These are not the immortal words that will set the world on fire, but they are the words of quiet heros, making their way day-by-day. From my perspective, one of the finest and kindest acts you can perform with another person is an honest, open, and simple conversation.

This is not easy to do. There is no adequate way to prepare for all the changes that occur in relationships when a chronic illness enters the picture.

"Prayer is the language of love. Different nations have different languages; love has its own language, no matter what nation we belong to. "

——ANONYMOUS

How can you explain your illness to the most important person in your life when you have just received the news yourself? Neither of you has a crystal ball to see the future. A chronic condition is certainly not in anyone's life plans.

Explaining your chronic illness to your significant other is like trying to predict the outcome of an automobile accident before it happens. No one can say whether you will walk away without a scratch or suffer a permanent disability. Or imagine that the doctor has just discovered you or your loved one has cancer. He can quote the survival statistics for that particular type of cancer, but he cannot predict until much later what the outcome will be for you. Of course, by then you've already lived through the worst of the uncertainty.

"One of the signs of maturity is a healthy
respect for reality—a respect that manifests itself
in the level of one's aspirations and in the
accuracy of one's assessment of the difficulties
which separate the facts of today from the bright
hopes of tomorrow. **"**

——ROBERT H. DAVIES

CHRONIC ILLNESS MEANS NEVER BEING ABLE TO SAY, "THIS IS FOR CERTAIN"

After being diagnosed, it may take more than just a few days or weeks for us to even begin to understand what disease we have, how to pronounce it, what its symptoms are, and how it may affect our lives. It took me a while just to learn to spell systemic lupus erythematosus, let alone understand how I was going to learn to live with it! My doctors could explain how my illness might act, but they couldn't predict the future for me.

You and your doctor can prepare yourself and your loved ones for potential changes, but at best, these will be general and quite vague. "You're going to be more tired," the doctor says, "so rest more often." What does that mean? No one seems to be able to tell you the important information, such as how long you can stay out of the hospital, how much your medical bills will total, or what kinds of activities you will or will not be able to do again.

After all the uncertainty we go through prior to the diagnosis, this can be very aggravating. As you begin experiencing daily frustration because of what you don't know, your relationships will be strained. You may begin hearing, "Aren't you better yet?" and "Why doesn't anyone know what's wrong?" from your heretofore supportive spouse. Try as you might, you may not get the long-overdue stability you both crave.

The "little surprises" thrown at you by your illness may keep you off balance for a long time. A hurry-up trip to the doctor, a spilled drink, a cancelled evening out with friends, an embarrassing moment with business associates, a disappointed child, a burned or never-made meal—these are the things that drive us crazy! Why can't our life run more smoothly?

"Wait a minute," you protest. "My Richard is a prince. He will always understand. I'm sure he will always be patient and supportive, like he is now." If this is true, Richard is not a prince, he's a saint! Most of us aren't lucky enough to have a St. Richard—or St. Joan of Arc, either. This is not a realistic view of any person, and it is dangerous because this attitude lulls us into a false sense of security. More likely, your Richard is struggling with his own doubts, fears, frustrations, and other feelings regarding your illness. When they finally do surface, they may be so complicated and strong that neither one of you can sort them out and deal with them without professional guidance.

Do yourself a favor, and initiate a few discussions with your spouse about your deeper feelings. Make it easy for him or her to talk, too. Don't put your partner in the awful position of having to transform himself or herself into a mind reader or highly skilled communicator overnight in order to accommodate your illness. It's not fair. Keep in mind that your spouse is the same person now as he or she was before you became ill. If your husband has always had a hard time telling you how he feels, or usually gets choked up when he says he loves you, you can expect him to have the same difficulties now. You may have begun to change first because your illness is closer to you, but he is the same person until you help him change.

By communicating early and often, you can avoid many of the problems before they begin. Talk—and listen—about anything and everything. Your illness certainly wasn't the only interesting part of your life together before you were diagnosed, so it shouldn't be after the diagnosis, either. Build upon the common interests and experiences that you share. Make it easy for your partner to be a successful supporter of your efforts, and remember to support his efforts as well.

Now is not the time to become selfish with your thoughts or "quality" time. Your parter needs you at your best, too, for all of those things you have provided in the past: An interested ear, a sounding board, a funny joke, a happy conversation, a warm hug, and all the rest. Continue striving to be your very best for each other, and the illness will not overwhelm either of you. Maybe it is bigger than both of you, but if you're smart and careful in your communication, you can beat your problems together.

EACH OF YOU WILL ADOPT NEW ROLES

Perhaps you will recognize some of the feelings and communication problems Betsy and Frank are going through:

Frank's chronic condition has kept him off the job for more than three months. He has been the primary wage-earner for the family, but at the present time, he is too ill to work. His job is being held open for him while he is on sick leave, but no one is sure for how long. It is uncertain if he will ever be able to go back to work.

Everything that he does is painful for him at this time. Getting out of bed and getting dressed, especially when buttoning or snapping are involved, are almost impossible. Each little motion that we take for granted causes him pain, and it may take half the morning just for him to care for himself, make breakfast, and clean up his dishes. He must rest frequently, as he has virtually exhausted himself performing his personal chores. His entire day continues in the same vein, and by the time his wife arrives home, he is exhausted, has extremely painful joints, and may be running a fever.

Betsy is privately trying to decide whether she should get a new job or increase the hours at her current job. She is worried: Can Frank take care of his physical needs at home?

How do you think her husband feels about this change? Not only is he hurting physically, but he is also trying to cope with the concept of being ill. He is also likely to be hurt because his wife is bringing home the bacon. His wife and doctor seem to be making all of his decisions. It's a frustrating, humiliating situation. It is probable that he will take his feelings of anger out on his wife or family.

Now imagine what Betsy is experiencing. She is working long hours, and then rushing home to care for her family's needs. She is still probably doing most of the cooking, cleaning, and shopping. She is beginning to feel resentful, and may take her feelings out on her husband, her children, her mother, or whoever else happens to be around. An honest and open discussion with Frank would probably help, but this is hard to do when feelings are already near the breaking point. Frank and Betsy both sense the need for better communication, but since neither of them have ever been through anything like this before, they are uncertain what they need and confused about how to get it. They are each adopting new roles, not entirely by their own choice, and thus they need new communication skills.

There is no mystery as to what they have to do. They must learn to talk to each other in new ways, ways by which they can clearly express their new thoughts and feelings. At the same time, they must also learn to listen and set their own feelings aside in order to support each other.

You know what it will sound like when Betsy, the quiet angel of mercy in Frank's life, finally has to say something to release the frustration building inside of her as she spouts:

"Honey, I feel so tired when I get home from work. I know that it's not your fault that you are ill, but it really hurts me to know that you are here and no one makes an effort to do laundry, straighten up the house, or start dinner. Don't you care how *I* feel? I can't take much more of this."

You can imagine how Frank will respond to this the first time he hears it. Now he feels guilty for being ill and putting his wife through so much hardship. The children, if they are old enough to hear and understand their mother's complaint, will also feel guilty because they played outside after school or went to a friend's house. Betsy may feel less frustrated, but she doesn't feel any better, as she has made everyone else miserable. All too often this is where the conversation ends. The communication process—and the healing process—has been started, but broke down before anything was accomplished.

Wouldn't it have been easier if she had said:

"Honey, I feel so tired when I get home from work. I know you can't do much right now because your illness is in a flare, but do you think that you could choose one chore you think you can handle and help me out by doing it?"

Ah, this is interesting: Betsy has expressed her frustration, and has taken it one step further by suggesting some action Frank could take that would help. Rather than blindly striking out at an aggravating situation, she has given him a "handle" on her part of the problem.

Now, Frank's no dummy. He knows Betsy well enough to recognize a big effort on her part to talk. He's feeling guilty enough as it is, so he jumps at the "handle" she's offering. It's not much, but it's enough to give him a couple of ideas:

> "I know how tough this whole illness thing has been on you. I really have been trying to do more, but maybe I'm not doing the right things. Rather than trying to catch up downstairs on the workbench, maybe I can do more for you."

Betsy is surprised to hear about the repair jobs he has been catching up on, and she softens a little. Her image of him sitting around the house all day feeling sorry for himself may be incorrect. Frank does a very smart thing at this point: He asks a question.

> "What bugs you the most when you come home?"

Betsy thinks for a moment, and explains that not having a clean kitchen to start dinner in drives her crazy. "It's hard enough to make dinner, and cleaning up just to get started puts me in a foul mood for the evening."

Frank quickly agrees that this is something he can do early in the day, before he runs out of energy. He mentally kicks himself for not seeing the problem earlier. "While I'm at it, maybe I could cook dinner." Betsy smiles and welcomes the help. "I know you hate to cook," she says, "but if you're willing to try, I am."

After a few more discussions and a couple of burned casseroles, they settle into a new routine that is more satisfactory. Frank still cleans the kitchen—in fact, he's become something of a neat freak—but he's taken over some of the laundry chores instead of the cooking.

The same lessons Frank and Betsy learned here applied to other aspects of their lives together. Frank wasn't able to attend all of their son's football games anymore, but he was able to spend more time helping him with his homework, and they enjoyed going to the movies together. He had to give up yard work altogether, but was able to plant a garden box. And Frank was able to take over an occasional PTA meeting and give Betsy an evening to herself.

Frank and Betsy had different problems, but they were rooted in the same cause. Because they both took the time to be specific and honest when they discussed their needs, they were able to negotiate solutions with which they could both live. With a few changes on both their parts, they are becoming more comfortable with their new roles and the new ways they relate to each other. They have to continue to work at it because they have no sense of permanency or normalcy yet, but they do have more confidence in their combined ability to cope with change.

> **"** Peace must be made. Like bread, it must be made daily. **"**
>
> ——G. Bromley Oxnam

NEW ROLES HAVE NEW NEEDS

Roles are likely to change in anyone's family when a crisis occurs. Roles will change automatically, but without discussion and forethought they will not change naturally. A woman who ran a house, and perhaps had a job as well, may now be a partial invalid and unable to work. Her status and esteem have changed and she has suddenly become the sick or "protected"member of the family. It's the same with the father who has been the chief wage earner. He finds household chores exhausting, and regrets that he never took time to develop any hobbies. His status and self-esteem plummet.

Just because a family lives together does not mean everyone intuitively knows about another person's needs. I can't read minds, and you probably can't either! But if we learn that it's all right to express our needs, and we learn a few effective ways to do it with our family, we will be able to protect and preserve our most valuable relationships.

We all have needs, and everyone around us has needs. My most acute need, right now, is to be acknowledged as a person, not as a victim of chronic illness. Also, I need hugs, lots of them, and as often as possible!

Now—today—is the time when everyone in the family has to sit down and have a talk about their own personal needs. It's a rude awakening for the family to realize the extreme variability of chronic illness; and it's a rude awakening for the person with the chronic illness to realize that he is not the only one with needs. Needs we all share are to be left alone sometimes, to talk out problems and find solutions, and to feel respected and needed, among many others.

There invariably seems to be a great deal of role changing going on soon after the diagnosis and throughout the first year of the illness. Each member of the family may shift into a different role in relation to the other family members. Who does what, and when they do it, are going to change anyway because of the natural maturation of your relationships with each other, but the chronic illness will accelerate this process.

I MISS BEING NEEDED

I miss being needed.
Once the whole family depended on me.
I was the breadwinner.
Only I didn't WIN the bread, I worked hard and earned it.
. . . I was needed at work.
In the community.
At home.
To build and haul.
To serve on committees.
To decide things.
To help people out.

——*Excerpted from*
GREEN WINTER, CELEBRATIONS OF OLD AGE

But, how do we make these changes work? Do we want interactions to be as they were before the illness was diagnosed? What is worth keeping, and what has to change? Did we have good communication before chronic illness entered the picture, or were we stuck in the complacent rut of non-communicative behavior? How do we make our most important relationships into whole, functioning units again? Here is what I've learned:

1. First, accept your "new norm," however humbling. If you can't accept yourself and respect yourself, why should anyone else?

2. Gain control of yourself, and resist the temptation to try to control others. They will have the same urge to control or fix the illness just because it seems so uncertain to them. "You look tired—why don't you rest now," and "You looked like you weren't interested, so I just assumed . . ." are signs that someone else is trying to control your illness. Your illness may be affecting them, but you are responsible for it and yourself.

3. Reinforce every person in the family so that each one knows how valuable he or she is to the family. Show each person active respect and insist that he do the same for the others.

4. Learn to sit down and face each other across the table and say "I need." We all have needs, but some people are reluctant to discuss their needs because they seem trivial in contrast to the magnitude of a chronic illness. It's far easier to deal with the needs of a relationship as they come up, because that's when they are most easily managed.

5. Develop new strengths. We are not as fragile as we think. If we give ourselves a chance to think about a problem from a new perspective, we can often tap resources and strengths that we may not have been using. Some of the "personal powers" that psychologists suggest we cultivate are mental power, will power, emotional (healing) power, physical power, social power, and spiritual power.

6. Play fair with yourself. Problems arise when we use our power to exert a negative influence because of the changes caused by chronic illness. For example, if we think of ourselves as victimized by chronic illness, our loved ones will quite naturally reinforce our attitude with unqualified support. They may adopt a protector role, perhaps even harboring a compulsion to take care of us because he or she sees the illness as a terrible threat to his or her happiness and security. Left unchecked, both of you may reinforce the negative, self-centered behavior of the other and each of you will lose a balanced perspective. Rather than letting the illness become the centerpiece of your relationship, make your relationship the centerpiece of your life.

7. Play fair with others. Take time to evaluate and forecast your illness often. Don't dwell on self pity, but rather make an intelligent determi-

nation of how your illness will behave, and communicate your best guesses to those around you. This will help those around you plan accordingly. Don't make a public announcement of your condition, and don't under any circumstances use your illness to manipulate or control others, but let them know what's going on clearly and honestly. All of those around me have said at one time or another: "No surprises, please!" There is no excuse for being sneaky about having your needs met. The better you become at predicting your energy level or activity level, the more they will trust you when you say you can or cannot participate.

8. Retain control and use the authority you have wisely. As a parent, be sure that each child is getting the time, love, and help he or she needs. Be willing to give away some authority. Your spouse, children, and others who are closest to you shared your goal to make the most out of your lives together before the diagnosis, and they still do, even if it means you relate to each other in different ways. This is for your own good as well as theirs. Don't try to fight change, but be selective and try to make the changes for the better. Allow outside help. Allow yourself the right to have a chronic illness. As time goes by, you should find yourselves settling into your new life together. It's like having a baby; life is never the same, but it can still be really great!

9. Restore equilibrium to your daily routines as quickly as possible. You will find that how you act has a definite influence on how others view you and how they act, too.

10. Be specific. State your needs without being coy or gruff. For example, instead of being grouchy and out-of-sorts when you get home from work, it might be easier if you just stated, "I am very tired this evening. Could you all help me by getting dinner started while I change?" This way, other people know just where they stand. They also are very likely relieved to know that your exhaustion and anger aren't from anything they have done. Your family and friends will be less fearful and confused if you state specifically what the problem is. If, for example, it is difficult for you to get out of a car, don't expect the driver to know about your problems. Instead, try telling him, "Jim, I can't lift my legs very well today. Could you help me by lifting them just a little and swinging them out?" Now, the driver knows precisely what to do to help you.

IT'S OK TO BE ANGRY: ACCEPTANCE IS AN ONGOING, FAMILY AFFAIR

Try as we might, we will never be able to communicate *completely* to those we love our frustration, pain, and sense of loss. It is our illness that is affecting them, not the other way around. Nevertheless, for them, like us, the chronic illness experience is maddening, uncertain, and frequently hard to understand.

Our illness will occasionally wreak havoc in our personal relationships, breaking down our health and self-esteem. Spouses or significant others will do the best they can to withstand the buffeting and aftershocks of our problems, but we should expect them to alternate between anger, sadness, and disbelief.

For a short period after the diagnosis, there is an almost childlike trust in one another. Married couples will exchange terms of endearment and pledge eternal love. The ill person receives promises of constant care and attention. All too often the spouse or other central person later finds these promises burdensome or impossible to fulfill.

The reality of our illnesses can take weeks and even months to understand even at the most basic levels. Uncertainty plagues us. Questions persist, no matter how much we know. How will I feel in five, ten, or twenty years? How will I function? How am I going to handle an illness that will last the rest of my life? We cling to the fantasy that somehow, in spite of what we know and what the doctor says, we will get back to where we were before.

Those around us take their cues from us, choosing to believe the unbelievable. Eventually, if all of us work hard at it, we resign ourselves to the realization that chronic illness is here to stay. We understand in our heads that somehow we and our loved ones have to change our lives and the nature of our relationships so we can get on with the rest of our lives. But we don't always understand that in our hearts.

Regrettably, those around us may not accept our illness at the same time, for they have to work through their own feelings. Many marriages and lifelong friendships do not survive.

This seems like the right time to confess that I have had a harder time writing this section than any other in the book. I would begin, tear it up, and begin again. Finally, when I stopped to analyze why I was having so much trouble, the answer hit me like a ton of bricks! My husband and I have had, and are still having, a very difficult time dealing with our anger at how our life has changed since I developed my illness. Even three years after the diagnosis, we are still having problems communicating about it. Writing about anger really hits close to home, but pehaps by sharing our problems, our experiences might give some insight—or warning!—to others dealing with similar feelings of anger.

Anger is not an emotion any of us particularly wants to face. Unfortunately, chronic illness inevitably arouses a tremendous amount of anger, both in the persons suffering from the illness and in those close to them. Those of us who routinely ignored or avoided angry feelings before can no longer afford to do so, now that they have become such a powerful and dominating force in our lives.

"Words can sting, but silence breaks the heart. "

—SEFRA PITZELE

Sometimes I think I have done a fairly good job of accepting my illness, yet I am constantly amazed that I still suffer moments of absolute fury. For months after my diagnosis, *I felt angry much of the time.* I am learning that I can only cope with my angry feelings by "owning" them. My anger is mine, and mine alone, and it is up to me to channel it or get rid of it.

I have a choice either to bend the ear of a sympathetic friend or professional, or to express my anger directly. When I do express anger, I try to zero in on a specific action or circumstance. For example, if I am exhausted beyond belief, and one of my children drops three eggs on the floor, my impulse is to immediately chastise the child. Instead, I have learned to acknowledge my exhaustion both to myself and to the child: "Don't worry about breaking the eggs. But could you please clean them up? I'm just too tired to help." In this way, I eliminate the reason for my anger, the mess on the floor, without making anyone feel ashamed or guilty.

One thing I have learned is that if I keep myself aware that I am getting angry, I can usually cope better. I remind myself that this is *my* anger, and since I own it, I have to try to take care of it first.

I have also developed my own warning signals, which let the family know that I am having a rocky time. Some of my favorite are *"This wouldn't be the best time* for you guys to pick at each other during dinner,'' and *''I'm too tired* to deal with this problem right now.''

Finally, I try to avoid reaching that state of total exhaustion which I call the point of no return. I am far more likely to flare up when my body is worn out. Slowly, but surely, I am learning to rest *before* I hit my point of no return.

❝ There are three things extremely hard: Steel, a diamond, and to know one's self. ❞

——MEGIDDO MESSAGE

In addition to my own anger, I have had to come to terms with my husband's feelings. I was in no way prepared to deal with the extent of my husband's anger. If one of our children or a friend became angry, I tended to distance myself from it a little more easily than if the anger came from my husband.

My husband, for the most part, is a patient and understanding man. And yet he continues to have a most difficult time dealing with my illness. The times when I have needed him to be the most understanding and demonstrative seem to be the times when he is most likely to be emotionally unavailable, or quick to express his anger. Other people I know have found themselves in similar situations with their loved ones. Either the person they care about the most totally ignores their pain or discomfort, or instead portrays anger that seems to be out of proportion to the situation.

In the beginning, I assumed that all my husband's anger was directed at me personally. I noticed that when I was obviously having a bad day or evening, he would quietly simmer for several hours, then erupt. I felt his anger personally and took refuge in silence and resentment. I was hurt and confused at his apparent lack of support and sympathy. After all, I reasoned, it was *my* illness; because I was the one who was suffering, I alone had the exclusive right to be angry. I was so busy passing judgment on my husband's behavior that I forgot, or perhaps chose to ignore, that he also had feelings and a different viewpoint.

Not wanting to cause conflict, I consciously limited what I said and when I said it. My husband, I thought, did not want to come home after a long day at work and hear all my complaints. Meanwhile, he was becoming equally careful about what he said and when he said it. Looking back, it seems so obvious: He learned that if he didn't ask me how I was, he wouldn't have to hear the answer and deal with either of our feelings. We were carefully not communicating. Anger was present for many months, but we did not deal with it at all. This continued until we finally realized what we were doing to each other.

It took many months for us to realize that his anger was not directed at me, but was, in fact, directed at the changes that this illness has caused in our lives and in our lifestyle. This is, I feel, the *key* to understanding anger among your loved ones as it relates to chronic illness.

We've spent many tearful and tormented discussions exploring our anger and frustration. I think this is close to the truth: My husband was not angry at *me*. He was angry because he felt *so totally out of control* with regard to my illness. He can't help me when I am hurting. He feels helpless. He can't really do anything for me to make me feel better, and so he becomes angry. He couldn't "kiss and make it better." Our life together—and our lives apart from each other—were being changed every day and he couldn't do a thing about it! This omnipresent illness was unplanned and unwanted. While I regarded my illness as an up and down process that changed daily, he saw only the negative side that never seemed to improve.

It has taken a great deal of time, patience, and understanding on both of our parts, but I finally realize that he has not been angry at me. He has been angry because of his sense of frustration, his fears, his feelings of helplessness, and his loss of my companionship during some of the evenings. Understanding why he is feeling so angry doesn't take the hurt away, but it *does* help each of us not to take it so personally and get angry in return.

WITH THE RIGHT COMMUNICATION SKILLS, YOU CAN KEEP YOUR RELATIONSHIPS GROWING

I don't intend for this to be an abbreviated marital relations course. But you must recognize early the heavy strain chronic illness can put on even the strongest relationships. It is urgently necessary for you to remain an adult, and replace whining, crying, and self-pity with new communication skills.

You and your loved ones need to sit down together and work at keeping your relationship the way you want it to be. Each of us has different needs, and each relationship has a uniqueness that makes it precious and worth protecting. Work together to find your comfort zones, and keep working together to keep them intact.

I wish that I had been forewarned. I wish I'd had more time to make right what was wrong between us. But my marriage is over now, and these were some of the reasons it ended. I wrote the following poem just after my husband asked me for our divorce.

OVER

I can see it in your eyes.
I can hear it in your voice.

We have struggled together.
Oh, how we tried to beat the odds
and make our marriage last.

No chance now for laughter,
only room for tears.

No more the dewy-eyed bride
ready to love and cherish,
only a mature woman who understands
your needs and your pain.

The odds were stronger than we were.
The spectre of my illness
was stronger than the bonds of our marriage.

And now you are gone.

—*SEFRA PITZELE, 1984*

Perhaps with an early awareness of the tremendous burden chronic illnesses or medical conditions place on loved ones, you can start working earlier on your relationships. No one can prevent a break up that is inevitable, but careful, early intervention that is rich with good communication skills may make the difference for you.

"BUT WHO WILL TAKE ME TO THE ZOO?"

Telling the children about your illness

Children who grow up with a parent who has physical limitations accept those limitations as a simple reality. When a child grows up with a parent who is blind or deaf, the child does not question the situation because he knows nothing else.

If a very young child has never known his parent to be anything but chronically ill, he will accept, as children normally do, that things in his home are "normal." At around three or four years of age, however, the child will begin to ask questions. They will range from "Why is Mommy (or Daddy) different from Timmy's Mom?" to "How come Dad can't walk?" to a frank "What's wrong with you, Mom?"

However, children whose parents have a newly diagnosed chronic illness have to make an adjustment to their new norms just like their parents.

During the time that the parent is suffering through the prodromal phase of illness, the child is usually suffering emotionally.

Much as we may want to shelter or protect them, our children are extremely vulnerable at this time. Concealing symptoms and discussing our concerns in whispered conversations with our spouses will not keep the illness a secret. Even young children are very intuitive. They know when something is wrong or about to change. They suffer more from the fear and tension of not knowing than they do from knowing the truth. We have no choice but to tell our children about our illness honestly and openly.

TO MY CHILDREN

When you were tiny, life was fine
A hug, a kiss, some milk, some time
A little nap and all aglow
Racing forth outside you'd go.

Life has changed now that Mom is ill.

Just know how much I love you, and know how much I care
And when you go to bed at night, we'll utter one small prayer.
Pray to gain your childhood back, unencumbered by my ill.
The way you have adjusted, my children, I am certain that you will!

——SEFRA PITZELE, 1984

Remember that children only want and need answers to that which they have asked. If, for example, a three-year-old asks her pregnant mother, "How does the baby get out?" all she really wants to know is that the birth canal (the vagina) stretches to open large enough to let the baby out when the baby is ready to be born. She doesn't need to know more than she has asked. The next time she asks, she will want more information. And next time, you can answer just a little more thoroughly.

This is also true of questions about chronic illness. For any age child, but especially for the child who is not yet old enough to attend school, simple answers are the best. A small child can be told, "Dad is in a wheelchair because his muscles won't work in his legs." A simple answer to a simple question! Say it with words they can understand, and give them the benefit of some explanation: "I can't work a puzzle with you now because my fingers are sore and won't bend, but I'd like to watch you do it and I'll help you choose the right pieces," is adequate for most small children. That much information is certainly better than, "No, not now."

But how do we explain something that we barely understand ourselves?

Those of you who have not yet told your children about your illness may find the following suggestions helpful.

Choose the time for telling your children carefully. You should be feeling well, or at least rested. If possible, your spouse should be present. Try to pick a time when your children are not tired or distracted by their own concerns. Make sure you tell all the children at the same time. There is less chance of misinterpretation or distortion if your children receive the same information from you. Also, your announcement will seem less frightening if the children are together to support and reassure each other.

You may find it useful to write down the name of your illness on a slip of paper. Reading the name of your illness can help your children become more familiar with it.

Try to tailor your explanations to the age level of your children. An approach that works with a young child will seem phony and patronizing to a teenager.

Children under the age of eight or so should be told only the most simple information. For example, if you have muscular dystrophy, you might say, "Sometimes I feel very tired, and my hands or legs are not strong. Sometimes I have to take naps in the afternoon, just like you do when we're going to a movie at night."

This explanation should be confined to the visible effects of the illness. You don't need to go into *why* you are tired and weak; your child will only feel helpless and burdened by information he can't understand. But he knows what he can see, and he can readily understand needing a nap as something familiar and reassuring.

Perhaps your children will react to your information with a lot of questions. Here are a few examples of questions commonly asked and some suggestions for answering them.

■ *"What will it do to you?"* "I really don't know for sure. It might get a little better with the new medicine I'm on. The doctor will help me."

■ *"What should I do to help you feel better?"* "If you can do some of the yardwork, that will help an awful lot. And maybe you can start carrying the garbage out to the garage."

■ *"Can you still work? Who will buy our clothes and stuff?"* "Right now, I can't work. But your Mom (or Dad) has a good job, and she can support us until I'm feeling well enough to work again. We might not be able to buy as much as we used to, but you'll always have clothes and enough to eat. Don't worry about that.''

Younger children generally have a short-term orientation. They have a very poor sense of time, and this is to your advantage right now. They are not as sensitive to the passage of time as you are, so they don't notice the gradual changes that you notice. Once they have accepted the basic fact of your illness, they will automatically accept all future changes.

CHANGES

Changes are something in life that everybody goes through.
Adjusting to a parent who has a chronic illness is
one of the hardest changes of all.
You don't understand the illness, but you do know
your whole life has changed.
Soon you begin to realize that it's really just the beginning.

It's so important to know that it's not
the end of the world, and life still goes on.
The sun still rises and the sun still sets, and love is like the
ocean, because even illness does not make it end.

So never let a cloudy day ruin your sunshine,
for even if you can't see it, the sunshine is still there,
inside of you, ready to shine when you will let it.

——*Amy Pitzele,*
9½ Years Old, 8/15/83

The question of death may come up frequently in your conversations with your younger children. They may ask repeatedly whether you are going to die, even after you have reassured them on this point. They may also display a great interest in death in general. "What happens to bodies when they are buried?" and "Do dead people get cold in the winter?" are typical questions. Don't let your children's apparent morbidness throw you. It is quite normal for children to display great curiosity about death. Your illness might have triggered their questions, but most children ask them sooner or later.

Once children realize that you aren't going to die and that many, if not all things will stay the same, their questions will shift to their own concerns. They might want to know if you can still fix dinner, take them to a movie, or drive them to school. Don't be hurt by what seems to be selfishness on the part of your children. Instead, look upon it as a positive sign that your children feel secure enough to express their natural feelings and concerns to you.

Let me end on a note of reassurance. Children are resiliant. You have enough time to make a few mistakes and correct them. Don't feel guilty because you developed a chronic illness and don't let your children make you feel guilty, either. By nature, children dwell on wellness, not illness. If you present your illness as only one part of your otherwise normal life, they will see it that way, too.

While young children are likely to be curious at first about the illness, teenagers may make it a point to "see no evil, hear no evil, and speak no evil." This isn't because they aren't worried and frightened. They are, but they also have their own special concerns about the illness.

One major concern is to fit in with their peer group. Having a parent with a chronic illness definitely sets them apart from their friends. They may feel anger at the parent for being ill; anger, in turn, provokes guilt and shame. Teenagers frequently react to their complicated emotions by trying to ignore the whole situation. They may even accuse you of "staging" your illness. While your teenager may be very cooperative about helping around the house, he or she may never tell his friends or teachers that something out of the ordinary is happening at home. They feel trapped in the resulting loneliness and isolation.

Don't be discouraged or offended if your teenager avoids the subject of your illness. Make an effort to provide information about your condition anyway. Do this in a factual, nonthreatening way, without expecting much feed-back or reaction. For example, you might leave a new book that deals with your specific illness on the coffee table.

Encourage your teenager to talk about his or her feelings about the illness.

Rest assured that underneath a pose of cool indifference, your teenager is probably harboring fear, unspoken questions, and probably anger. You may want to bring up the subject by letting him know that you realize it's been hard and that it's okay to feel angry. Still, being angry is no excuse for poor behavior. It wasn't before your illness, and it isn't now. Try to make it easy for him to say ''I'm scared,'' ''I need a hug,'' and ''I love you'' (or ''I hate you''). They will appreciate your efforts to communicate with them, though they may not admit it. Adolescents are especially volatile emotionally. They can be ''up'' and ''down'' in a period of minutes. Do not take it personally, but if you feel you are the cause of a mood change, just ask. They'll tell you—loud and clear!

Older children in their late teens and twenties may be more independent, but they still need a great deal of reassurance. Keep in mind, however, that they are adults. You should be prepared for tough, detailed questions. Some will concern your illness:

■ ''How does the doctor know for sure that you have this disease?''

■ ''What kinds of tests did he do?''

■ ''Will you have to go into the hospital again?''

■ ''Are you certain he is the right doctor for you?''

Other questions might deal with their concerns about changes in their lives:

■ ''Is it hereditary?''

■ ''What is the mortality from this illness?''

■ ''Will you still be able to help me pay for school, or will I have to cover all my own expenses?''

Though your children may have many questions, don't try to be the ''perfect parent'' and pretend that you have all the answers. If they sense that you are hedging or concealing something, they will look for the answers on their own. You may find it easier to give your adult children something to read about the illness, particularly if you are not very familiar with it yourself. Remember, to children of any age, the most bitter truths are easier to deal with than the anxiety and uncertainty of not knowing.

Finally, emphasize to all your children that you are still learning about the condition yourself. You may need to have a number of discussions with them as you learn and understand more about it. Remember to show your concern for their feelings and worries. They need to know that their problems are as important to you as your illness is to them.

YOUR CHILDREN WILL NEED TO GRIEVE

Like each of us and like our spouses, children suffer losses that can only be healed by experiencing the grieving process. Soon after you have told your children, they will probably begin their grieving process. It is important for them to grieve, as it will help them accept the many changes that will take place in their lives.

Most of the changes caused by your illness will be counted as losses by your children. Medical bills may leave less money for food, clothing, or education. If you are forced to move because of the illness, your children will suffer additional upheaval. They may have to assume responsibilities that you can no longer handle. You and your children may no longer be able to participate together in active sports such as baseball, hunting, or skiing.

We must allow them to work through all the stages of grief, including anger. We must be prepared to hear things like, ``I hate you!'' or ``You're not sick! You just don't want to play with me!'' Anger from our loved ones hurts, but it helps to remember that our children aren't angry at us, they're angry because of their own pain and stress at the situation caused by the illness.

THEY STILL NEED YOU IN YOUR FAMILY ROLE

Maintaining as much of a normal family life as possible will help your children adjust more easily to your illness. Children depend on routines, so try to set up new ones that provide the same fun, warmth, and security as the old ones.

Illness may rule out some activities, but with a little imagination, families can discover equally satisfying substitutes. For example, ice fishing may take the place of skiing. Instead of taking long cross-country trips, consider substituting day excursions to local parks and cultural events. It may simply be a question of emphasis—more spectator sports and movies, less sandlot softball.

A little common sense and planning can lessen the impact of chronic illness on day-to-day family life. If everyone is looking forward to a child's ball game or bowling, you may want to avoid activities like cleaning the house or sweeping the garage that day. Keep your priorities straight! By conserving your strength, you may be able to participate in the outing as planned. Your children depend on you, and these types of activities are more important than your short-term sense of accomplishment.

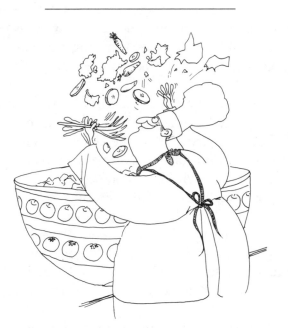

Jim tossed illness aside and tossed salad instead!

Sometimes, in spite of careful planning, changes have to be made. Symptoms can fluctuate just like the weather. Your child's slumber party may have to be cancelled because you aren't feeling well enough that day. An eagerly anticipated picnic may fall through because of your illness. When this happens, try to arrange an acceptable substitute. You can organize a family game of Monopoly, or your child can ask a friend to sleep over another day. If the child just wants to be left alone to accept the loss, that's okay, too.

SET A GOOD EXAMPLE

Probably the best way to help your children is for you to learn to adjust to your illness as well as you can. If you accept disappointments calmly and maturely, your children will follow your example. You and your spouse should attempt to present a stable, united front to the children in spite of any misgivings or confusion about the illness. Tensions between the two of you can seriously hinder your children in their efforts to cope. Unless you come to terms with the illness, you cannot expect your child to do so. If you or your spouse presents an image of being continually overwhelmed and consumed with self-pity, don't be surprised if your children either resent you or imitate you.

The child can react to tension in the parents' relationship in the following ways:

■ Behaving well at home, but acting up in public.

■ Waiting until you are very tired before making a personal demand such as, "You have to show me how to shoot baskets. The gym teacher said I had to learn."

■ Overtly lying about the situation. ("My Mom is going to die next week.")

■ Regressing to more childlike behavior.

■ Trying out a contrived illness to see how much sympathy he can get.

■ Throwing temper tantrums or expressing anger in another socially unacceptable way.

■ Announcing that he can't possibly go to school because he is "too tired."

■ Crying at night or suffering from sleeping problems or nightmares.

I should add that some children practice these manipulative techniques even when their parents adjust well to the illness. Any major change or stress is enough to set them off. *If a child continues to display negative and manipulative behavior over a long period of time, consult a professional!* Don't assume that the problem will eventually disappear. We must remain sensitive to any changes of behavior in our children. Our illness is going to create enough difficulties for the whole family. We don't have to add to our problems by ignoring a child's need for help until it is too late.

Remember to be a good parent. Before you became ill, your children knew the house rules and were expected to obey them. The same should hold true now. Your illness—or anyone else's, for that matter—is not an excuse to relax discipline, look the other way, or make special allowances. Kids need a predictable home life, and your job is to give it to them.

" Do not judge a man until you have walked in his moccasins seven days. **"**

——INDIAN PRAYER

KEEPING YOUR FRIENDSHIPS GROWING

During the early phases of our illness, many of us came to depend on the support of our closest friends. They stood by us faithfully. They were among the few who realized how much pain and discomfort we were suffering behind our facade of normality. Without being asked, they stepped in and ran errands or did yardwork when we were too ill to manage. They helped not only when they were feeling in a generous mood, but when helping was difficult or inconvenient. Those of us who have been blessed with friends like this will always be grateful to them.

Sooner or later, we will stop viewing chronic illness as the dominant influence in our lives, and we must ask or give permission so that our friends do the same. We must emphasize to them that although our bodies and physical abilities have changed, the shared thoughts, feelings, and interests that created the friendship still remain. We need to let them know that we want to have a two-way friendship again, where we give as well as receive.

❝One good friend is worth a hundred psychiatrists. ❞

——SEFRA PITZELE

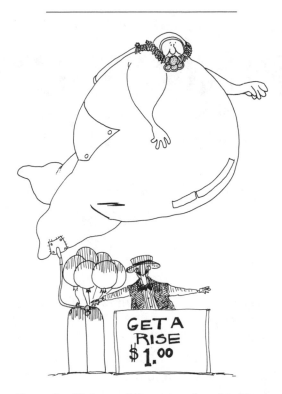

Howard will do anything to rise above his illness.

The following guidelines can help you put your friendships back on a more equal footing.

1. Don't leave your friends in the dark. If they express an interest in learning more about your illness, explain it to them. Perhaps you can share some of the literature you've been reading.
2. Don't hesitate to ask your friends for help or to take advantage of their offers. Make certain, however, that you are not wearing out their generosity. If your needs require a great deal of time and attention, you may find it necessary to hire outside help, such as a home health aide or community volunteer. Over-dependence on friends can create unnecessary tension and guilt.

"A friend is a person with whom I may be sincere. Before him, I may think aloud. "

—RALPH WALDO EMERSON

3. Your friends may sometimes unintentionally come across as overbearing or condescending. For example, they may say, "Let me get that door for you. It doesn't look as if you can manage it." Don't be offended. Remember that they mean well, even though they don't always express themselves in the most tactful way. A simple, "Thanks, but I think I can do it," is the best and clearest response.

4. Don't be afraid to discuss that status of your friendship openly, particularly if you sense that your illness has changed your friend's feelings toward you. Out of concern for your well-being, your closest friends may tend to concentrate on your illness to the point of forgetting everything else.

COMPROMISE

Life is a series of compromises
In which we all must bend
But knowing that we want to share
Will help us reach the end.

—SEFRA PITZELE, 1982

5. Make an effort to participate in social activities. Let your friends know that although your activities are limited by your illness, you can still be involved. Be flexible and think of acceptable substitutes for activities that you can no longer participate in. For example, if you can no

longer play tennis, maybe you can get together with your friend to watch a tennis match on television. Or totally change the type of activity you do together. Try a concert or movie, go shopping together, or organize a potluck dinner.

6. If you are physically disabled and are planning an evening with a friend at a theater or restaurant, call ahead to make sure the building is accessible. Express this need to your friend, and perhaps he or she can help you make suitable arrangements. A bit of preplanning will help you avoid embarrassing situations that draw attention to your physical condition and perhaps cast your friends in unexpected and uncomfortable roles.

❝ The best mirror is an old friend. ❞

—JACULA PRUDENTUM

7. Listen to yourself carefully to make sure that you are not dominating conversations with the subject of your illness. Remember that you and your friend do need to talk about it, but not all the time. Both of you will benefit if you continue to take an interest in other things.

8. Don't forget to ask your friend how he or she is doing. Remember, you have an equal obligation to take an interest in your friend's concerns.

❝ If you don't lose your mind over certain things, you have no mind to lose. ❞

—JOHANN NESTROY

With your acquaintances and more casual friends, you may encounter credibility problems. Because your contact with them tends to be brief and superficial, they are less likely to see beyond the deceptively healthy facade that often hides a chronic illness. They cannot believe that you are seriously and incurably ill. They assume that because you don't *look* sick, you *aren't* sick. On your worst days, you may hear comments like, "You look just wonderful! I'm so glad that you're feeling better!"

The same people frequently spread their own mistaken perceptions among *their* friends: "Have you seen Judy lately? She seems to have recovered from her bout of illness and she looks great!" Slowly but surely, your reputation for blooming health grows and the credibility gap widens.

What I have dubbed the "Paying the Piper" syndrome further complicates our credibility problems. Friends who see you out on the town enjoying yourself, attending a party, or holding down a job often don't realize the price you pay to do these things. You may only be capable of doing your job if you take a rest break every hour. A party or a night out may require a day in bed beforehand to rest up and a day in bed afterward to recover. Credibility does indeed suffer when people see only one side of your activities.

OSCAR

How am I doing? Fine, thank you.
I have become the great pretender, and I bet you pretend more often
than you'd like, too.

No one puts on a show better than someone with a chronic illness.
Give us all Oscars.

——*Sefra Pitzele, 1983*

How do you correct the misperceptions of casual friends and acquaintances? I have learned that I am probably better off not doing any correcting at all. Attempts to regain full credibility with *everyone* I know are futile and self-defeating. If I spent my time trying to explain my true situation to them, I would bore my friends and myself.

When my casual friends ask me how I am doing, I recognize that they are not really asking about the state of my health. They are simply engaging in a polite social ritual. I usually say something like, ''I'm fine. Thank you for asking.'' While this may not be strictly true, this kind of reply is all that they need or want.

You may think that I am adding to rather than solving my credibility problems. But sometimes a few "white lies" about our condition are in order. We have a right to our privacy. We have a right to choose whom to tell, what to tell, and when to tell. The complete information may not fit a particular situation, and we have the freedom to make such judgments.

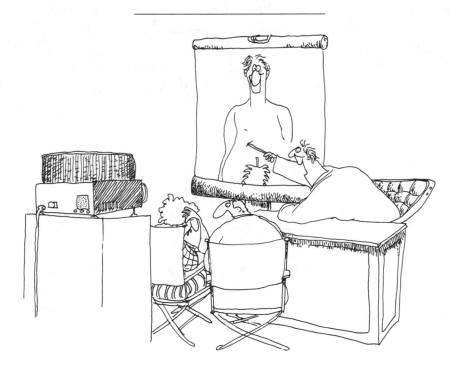

How not to explain your medical condition.

Up to this point, I have concentrated on existing friendships, both close and casual. But don't forget the joy and excitement of making new friends. Coping groups and associations of people who share your condition, community groups, or religious activities offer many opportunities to meet people. We all grow from each new friendship that we form.

In the end, your illness need not damage your new or existing friendships. Value your close friends for their faithfulness and loyalty. Enjoy the company of your casual friends, while accepting their more limited understanding of your condition. Make new friends at either level of intimacy. Most important, continue to be a loyal, sympathetic, and affectionate friend.

I'd like to close this chapter with some thought *for your friends*. You may wish to share this section with them, or just keep it in mind as your friendships grow and change.

To the friends of a chronically ill person:

■ Give your friend patience and empathy, but not sympathy. *Empathy*, in this context, means putting yourself in the other person's position in order to understand how he may feel. *Sympathy* means to feel sorry for them.

■ While sympathy may be a heart-felt expression which keeps a person going in a troubled time, it is up to each of us to keep sympathy from becoming pity.

■ Imagine yourself in the position of the person (or the family) who needs help. Perhaps, during a bad time, your friend is bedridden. What would help you if you were in bed all day?

PAIN

Pain isolates.
No matter how many friends you have
Or how well devoted.

——GREEN WINTER, CELEBRATIONS OF OLD AGE

■ Try to become educated about your friend's illness or medical condition. If you feel uncomfortable about asking your friend directly, call or write the local association for that specific problem or go to the public library. I must caution you, however, that if you do go to the public library, be sure that the information you are reading is from current literature. More than one person has been panicked by out-of-date information.

■ Perform whatever actions you feel will help the person or the family. An example is to cook dinner and take it over, or help with the grocery shopping or chores.

■ Don't make idle offers. Even if your intentions are excellent, don't offer unless you are really willing to carry through.

■ Don't leave offers open-ended. Regardless of your sincerity, don't put the burden of asking for help solely on the shoulders of the person who needs the help.

■ If you're not sure what to do, follow your own instincts about how to act. Even if you are not very close to the person with the medical problem and you feel like making an encouraging phone call, go ahead and do it. More than one new friendship has begun because someone showed he cared. Make that first step.

■ Be especially tolerant of your friend until the initial adjustment to chronic illness has passed. Remember, he has just lost his good health and he needs time to grieve.

■ Never talk down to a person who has a chronic condition. He can still think, feel, and make decisions. Look at the examples below, and then listen to yourself the next time you talk to your friend with the illness.

You might say something like: "Let me get that door for you. You sure can't do it yourself."

It would be better to say: "Can I help by getting the door?" Then wait for an answer to your question.

You may say: "I'll go to the store for the groceries. You stay here and rest."

A better way to say it might be: "Let's go to the store together. If you get too tired, we can always come home."

■ Help your friend develop his "new norms" by treating him as a person, illness notwithstanding.

■ Be sure to level with your friend if there is a problem with your relationship. Be honest and tactful. For example:

"John, I'm having a problem with your attitude toward me since you got sick. I'm sure you don't mean it, but it seems that all you have needed me for recently is to run your errands. There's more to our friendship than that."

■ Include your friend in social plans, even if you feel the activity may be too tiring or otherwise inappropriate. Let your friend make up his mind about whether to accept. He may not be able to participate in the same way you do, but it is likely that he will still enjoy the time spent with friends.

■ Do not decide ahead of time what the other person can and cannot do. Chronic illness is so variable that a person's abilities may change quickly, perhaps even overnight.

■ It's not taboo to ask about your friend's health. It's a normal and comfortable part of friendship and very much expected. To never ask would be to ignore an important part of your friend's life.

■ Never assume that because your friend chooses not to talk about his illness (some people never mention it) that it has gone away. Chronic illness never goes away, although the effects will vary over time.

■ Remember that anyone, including those who have chronic illness, can have other crises in their family. Friendship is needed then in a special way.

■ Bear in mind that you are not performing a service by being a friend. Friendship is mutual, and both parties should gain from it.

DEAR FRIEND

Please do not think of me as an illness
Try not to forget that I still remain me.
Guide us both by dwelling upon my wellness
In order to help me set my own self free.

Though my body may not always respond to my commands
And my chronic illness makes its own constant demands,
I can still be a wife, mother, lover, or friend
If just a little you will bend,
To accommodate yet a different side
So that our relationship can still abide.

Take me as I take you, just for what I am.
I may look or act differently, but I'm doing the best I can.

I may walk more slowly and sometimes am in pain
But I'm still the same old person who loves walking in warm rain.
So walk with me now and try to hold my hand
And I will draw some strength from you because I know I can.

I never choose my friends for how they appear
But for loyalty, for solidness, for caring, and for cheer.

So let us hold hands my dear friend
And we'll smile and we'll cry and we'll share
And we'll bend
To accommodate the changes from which no one is exempt.
Being merely mortals we all each need the other
And I intend to guard our friendship as if you were my brother.

I love you dear friend
For being there and caring
So let's dwell on my wellness,
On our doing, living, sharing.

Bless you for being there through thick and through thin,
For we know the deep importance of how friends
Can help us win.
Sometimes we don't know we've fought the battle
Until we've won the war,
And friendship, love, and giving are what the world is for.

——*SEFRA PITZELE, 1983*

YOUR HEALTH CARE TEAM

Y ou probably never planned to have your association with your doctor become a complicated, give-and-take relationship. By the one-year anniversary of your diagnosis, it is likely that you will know if she has children, when she goes on vacation, what time she arrives at her office each day, and great deal more personal information.

Your doctor will likewise know a lot more about you a year from now. Regardless of the type of relationship you had before your diagnosis, you, your doctor, and many other medical professionals are now partners in your health care. Your shared goal is to keep you as well and as mobile as possible.

The quality of your relationship with your doctor can make the difference between a well-managed illness and needless pain or inconvenience. Like a marriage, this is a complex relationship that merits extra time and effort.

Rabbi Bernard Raskas puts it this way:

No gain without pain: "In the techniques that modern medicine uses to treat people, progress is made only at the price of persistent strain. In physical rehabilitation we have to stretch the muscles in order to gain full use of them. In dealing with mental illness, we often have to face painful emotions and insights in order to find the way toward healing relationships.

These examples show us that the path to proper living is not strewn with roses but filled with rocks that have to be lifted out of the way. And even when there are roses along our path, when we reach to pick them we may be stuck with thorns and have to pause to pull them out of the flesh.

A physician once prescribed some pills for a young patient. The pills were coated with sugar to make them palatable. When the youngster failed to show any improvement, the puzzled doctor asked the mother whether the child had taken the medicine regularly. The mother was determined to watch her son when he took the pill. She noticed that the lad licked off the sugar coating with his tongue and then threw the pill down the drain. Now she understood why her child was not getting better.

Accepting only the sugar-coated parts of life and avoiding its bitterness will not yield strength. But, if we are willing to accept the pressures and the struggles along with the joys, we will live a healthy and successful life. Life will be good if we determine that, no matter what, we will achieve our worthiest and most honorable goals. Given this commitment, we will learn that the real miracle of existence is not what God does for us, but rather what God inspires us to do for ourselves and others in spite of the pain and strain.''

WHICH DOCTOR IS RIGHT FOR YOU?

Think about your doctor. Do you feel comfortable with him or her? Are you confident that you are getting the attention and care you need? Does he or she anticipate your problems and initiate solutions to the degree you would like? Is your relationship effective at problem-solving? Are you making progress?

It is nice, but not always possible, to stay with the same doctor before and after your diagnosis. Recognize that you are going to have different needs in the coming years. If you have generally been healthy and have not required much medical attention until recently, you have essentially an untested relationship that may need some additional thought and discussion.

The most important expectations we have concern our doctor's credentials. We should be certain that we are seeing a well-recommended family practitioner or a specialist who is qualified to care for our chronic illness. It amazes me that some people spend more time shopping for a car or a stereo system than selecting a doctor! I suggest that you ask your doctor directly how many other people like yourself he has treated. How does he feel about a long term relationship with your case? Does he feel professionally capable, or would he prefer to recommend you to a colleague with more practical experience?

Doctors with whom you have long-term relationships serve as diagnosticians and healers. They should help you prioritize your problems, and identify which need attention first. Your doctor should also be your liaison to all of the other medical services you will need to deal with your illness. It is your doctor who will send you to a consultant or a specialist (I have described most types of specialists on pages 44 to 47), and it is also your doctor who will decide when you need to add a therapist, nutritionist, or other person to your health care team.

WHAT CAN YOU EXPECT OF YOUR DOCTOR?

Whether he is a family practitioner or a qualified specialist, you can expect your physician to do his job: Keep you as healthy as medically possible. His professional objectivity requires a certain measure of distance, but this should not be confused with indifference. You need to feel that your doctor cares about you. You should feel that you can trust your doctor and that you are welcomed as an important member of your own health care team.

Other expectations must also be met if you are to get the care you need. Your doctor should show you kindness and empathy. You can expect that your physician will always be truthful with you. Sometimes the truth hurts; but surprises and suspicions that result from trying to conceal the truth are far more painful. Similarly, he can expect you to be truthful in return. Doctors can't read minds. They can't even try to solve a problem you don't tell them about! Once you have shared your problem with your physician, you can expect him to act upon it in one way or another, even if it is to reassure you that nothing serious is wrong.

You can expect your doctor to be as open and truthful with your family as he is with you. He should be willing to help them understand your medical condition, or to help you properly explain it to them.

You can expect your doctor to show his care for you by giving you his full attention while consulting with you on the phone or during an examination. The doctor allots a certain length of time for your visit; that time is yours exclusively. It should not be spent answering the phone, seeing other patients, or talking to the office staff.

You can and should expect your physician to be human. If he is late for an appointment or out of sorts, avoid taking it personally. He may have had a long night on call, or he might not be feeling well himself. You must remember that doctors have families and problems just like the rest of us. They aren't immune from illness, either.

CRITERIA FOR SELECTION

Here is a short checklist to keep in mind as you evaluate your present doctor or think about selecting a new physician:

1. *He should be board certified.* If he isn't, he may not have been exposed to suitable training. Certification is no guarantee of superior care, but the absence should give you pause. To find out, you can ask him, contact your local medical society, or look him up in the *Directory of Medical Specialists* or the *Directory of Physicians in the U.S.* Also find out where he did his residency, the two or more years of training and working after medical school. University-affiliated hospitals are best.

2. *He should be aware of new developments.* Does he refer to recently developed treatments? Does he attend special conferences? Has he kept pace since he left medical school?

3. *He should be a member of his medical society.* Again, there are no guarantees, but a membership says something about peer review, and that's better than nothing.

4. *He should take time with you.* A doctor should diagnose *and* reassure you. Impatience or a harried demeanor discourages open discussion. Look for quality time when you can get your doctor's full attention. (Believe it or not, there are courses that teach doctors how to rush huge numbers of people through their offices each day. These courses are expressly designed to minimize time and maximize profits!)

5. *He should not be afraid of a second opinion.* Don't be afraid to ask for a recommendation if you are unconvinced or uncertain about a treatment. His reaction to your request will tell you much about his confidence in his diagnosis. If your doctor balks when you say you want a second opinion, seriously reconsider your relationship with him.

6. *He should admit when he's uncertain.* No one is perfect. For your part, make it easy for him to be open and frank.

7. *He should be a good communicator.* Does he speak in language you understand? Does he know how to "actively listen"? If you don't understand him, find someone else.

8. *He should be interested in you as a whole person, not just a clinical problem.* Again, this requires a trusting relationship that takes time to build.

WHAT YOUR DOCTOR EXPECTS FROM YOU

In turn, you as a patient have certain obligations to your physician. Here is a list of *Dos* and *Don'ts* for your relationship with your physician:

DOS

1. Be prepared for your office call, especially if it's for a new reason.
2. Follow the instructions you are given prior to the office visit (e.g., not eating before a blood test).
3. Make a list of the questions you want answered.
4. Take pencil and paper so you can write down and understand what he says.
5. Arrive for your office visit on time.
6. Insist that your doctor speak to you in language you can understand.
7. Speak to your doctor about *all* your concerns, no matter how small they seem.
8. Report any physical changes or drug reactions to your doctor.
9. Allow your doctor to send you to a consultant if necessary.
10. Advocate for yourself. If you hear of a new medical advance on TV or read about one in the newspaper, ask your doctor if it's pertinent to your situation.
11. Take empty medicine bottles or the drug names and prescription numbers to your appointment in order to facilitate the refilling of prescriptions.
12. Follow your doctor's orders exactly. If you don't understand or forget the instructions, *ask*.
13. Be willing and prepared to talk to the on-call physician if it's necessary.
14. Recognize that your physician needs to be paid for his services. Work out a plan to pay for office visits and complete any insurance paperwork promptly.
15. Believe in yourself. If you are convinced something is wrong, you are likely to be correct.

DON'TS

1. Don't insist on an immediate appointment if it's not an emergency.
2. Don't be angry if the doctor is "running a little behind" (15–30 minutes).
3. Don't feel you have to stay if he is *very* late. You have the right to reschedule your appointment.
4. Don't try to become too familiar with your doctor or call him by his first name. Doctors need to maintain their objectivity.
5. Don't waste your valuable appointment time with conversation that is not relevant to your medical condition.
6. Don't answer, "Fine," when the doctor asks how you are feeling. This meaningless answer forces your doctor to conduct a verbal investigation to find out what is wrong with you.
7. Don't lie to or mislead your doctor about anything. You are only harming yourself.
8. Don't feel hurt if your doctor has to refer to your chart to refresh his memory. After all, he has many patients and does not want to make an error.
9. Don't be modest. Doctors have seen bodies in all shapes, sizes, and conditions.
10. Don't expect your doctor to perform a complete physical during a short office visit. Physicals must be scheduled in advance.
11. Don't make any modification to your medicine dosage or schedule according to how you feel that day. Even if you are feeling better, medicine *must* be taken as directed.
12. Don't *ever* share your medicine with someone else, even if their symptoms seem identical. Not only is it very dangerous, but it is also a violation of federal law.
13. Don't make a call to the "on-call" physician for a minor problem that can be addressed during your doctor's regular office hours.
14. Don't ever feel uncomfortable for going to the doctor with what seems to you to be a "little" problem. He'll make that judgment.
15. Don't call for prescription refills after office hours.
16. Don't insist that the receptionist or nurse let you talk to the doctor unless it is an emergency. In that case, clearly state, "This is an emergency," and they will take the appropriate actions.

17. Don't cancel your appointment at the last minute unless it's absolutely unavoidable. Some physicians also impose a charge for appointments cancelled less than 24 hours in advance.
18. Don't speak to your doctor about a medical problem if you bump into him away from his office (like at the supermarket!).

Finally, your doctor needs to trust you for good feedback on which treatment is working and which treatment is not working. If his solution is ineffective, he wants to be the first to know. Would you still take an antibiotic until the bottle is empty if it gave you terrible stomach cramps or an upset stomach? Would you continue taking pills if you got a rash all over your body? Of course not. I hope you would call your doctor and explain the problem.

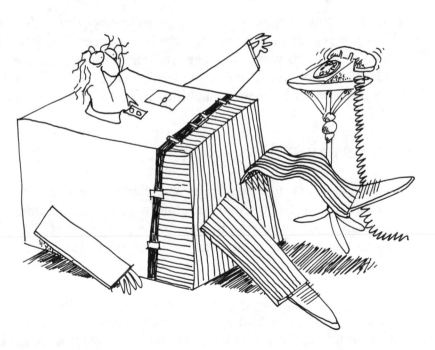

If minor side effects persist, consult your physician.

DEPENDENCY IS NORMAL

There is a normal tendency for a patient to become very attached to his physician immediately after a chronic illness is diagnosed. After all, the doctor represents the authority figure with the power to heal.

Primary care doctors who treat patients with chronic illnesses expect and understand this dependence. No phone call is "too silly" and no question is "too small" to answer. It is a part of their responsibility to you.

This pronounced dependence upon your doctor is often cyclical. It happens shortly after the diagnosis and during and after a frightening flare-up. Remember, this is normal and acceptable. Your life is changing, your body is unpredictable, and your trust in yourself has taken a beating.

You may feel that your doctor is literally your lifeline. It's okay to feel scared and uncertain, and to feel you really *need* him, especially in the beginning.

You and your doctor are partners. You need each other. You are his patient, and he is your advisor. He owns the medical degree, but you own the illness. You have to learn to work together and communicate clearly if your condition is to ever improve. I guesstimate that the best doctor/patient relationships are made up of 50% medical ability and 50% communication and mutual trust.

TRUST MUST BE EARNED

We trust our doctor because he's more knowledgeable about our illness than we are, particularly in the beginning before we have had a chance to get involved in our health care program. In fact, some people trust their doctors too much, even to the point of abdicating their responsibility to themselves. Don't depend completely on your doctor just because he's available.

You can expect your doctor to automatically distrust you for awhile. Until you prove otherwise, he is probably going to expect you to behave like most patients with an acute problem: You will do what he says for a short time, but as soon as you begin feeling better, you will do what you want instead. He will also expect you to have difficulty explaining all your symptoms at first.

Your doctor has to learn to trust you. Just like everyone else, you will have a short honeymoon period in which your forgetfulness and excuses will be tolerated, but eventually you will have to earn his trust by your actions.

THE ISSUE IS COMPLIANCE

The issue of compliance is probably already a sore point with your doctor. Patient noncompliance may be one of his most frustrating problems. He's learned that people generally do not follow "doctor's orders." He expects the same problem with you until you prove otherwise.

Compliance means to follow a prescribed treatment regimen as instructed by your doctor or another professional on your health care team. No matter how successful your medication or examination seems to be, it is your responsibility to stick to your program after you leave the doctor's office.

The consequences of noncompliance are serious. Failing to follow your doctor's instructions can cause serious complications of your condition, expensive hospitalization, greater pain, or other medical problems. Failure to take an antibiotic at the prescribed intervals, for example, can permit a strong organism to multiply unchecked, and can result in a more serious infection than you had initially. Similarly, unwillingness to comply with dietary recommendations to lower your salt intake or avoid certain foods can precipitate digestive disorders, allergic reactions, heart problems, and worse.

According to recent surveys, in spite of stern reminders from their physicians, more than half of all patients fail to follow instructions. They are more likely to comply if their episode is serious, less likely as they start to feel better. Most patients can follow a twice-a-day prescription better than a four (or more)-times-daily dosage. Not surprisingly, the compliance rate falls off rapidly with more complicated treatment programs. You may recognize some of these examples:

1. You forgot to take your medicine at lunch so you took it at three-thirty. Then it was too soon to take your dinner pill, so that got bumped, too. Now you have had only ¾ of your daily medicine.
2. The doctor tells you not to drink, but you give in one evening and have two martinis. After a short while, your stomach starts to give you incredible pain. Now you are faced with the awkward predicament of telling your doctor the truth in order to get some relief.
3. You used all your blood pressure medicine, but since you were going to see the doctor in a week, you decided to wait. Now you find yourself in the emergency room with very high blood pressure and a severe headache.

4. There wasn't enough money for your medicine so you didn't take *any* for several days. Now you realize what a predicament you may be in and you are too embarrased to call your doctor.

When pain or other symptoms return, the patient is reminded to get back on the program. Hopefully, it's not too late, but some "silent" diseases like high blood pressure do their damage without noticeable discomfort or symptoms.

Most doctors seem to want to say to their patients: "Look, I'm doing my best to keep you healthy. I expect you to do your best for yourself, too."

Doctors are human. They expect to have the problems listed above presented to them many times during the day. Generally, they will try to take the time to explain why it is so important to take medicine and other prescribed therapy with a chronic illness or medical condition. Generally they will do what they can to help you.

We've discussed compliance and how important it is. Now, I'd like to temper that view with a word of caution against blind compliance: If you notice any changes for the worse after beginning a new treatment, call your doctor immediately. Your doctor's orders may be wrong for you, but let him make that determination.

Because so many patients prove themselves to be poor compliers, your doctor may assume you will not follow instructions, either. Regardless of your previous relationship or compliance record, you must demonstrate that you are a dependable member of your health care team.

In order to comply with your doctor's instructions, you must feel *in control* of your illness and treatment program. The more you know about your illness, the more you should want to know about your treatment. If you understand why you are being asked to take certain medications, you are much more likely to comply. If the treatment makes sense to you, you are more likely to comply. You are ultimately responsible for your own comfort, health, and well-being.

While not every doctor appreciates this concept of patient authority and responsibility, most believe that patients should have more decision-making power. If you assert yourself a few times and then follow through with good compliance and good feedback on your doctor's recommendations, he should come around to your way of thinking. You both must trust each other to be working for the same goal: To keep you as healthy and as active as possible.

TRUST IS A TWO-WAY STREET

Your doctor will have to earn your trust, too. Unfortunately, doctors occasionally let their patients down. Has this ever happened to you?

"This is Mrs. Bateman. I am Dr. Anderson's patient. I have rheumatoid arthritis and am having acute pain in one knee. Would you please have the doctor call me?"

"Certainly, Mrs. Bateman. The doctor will call you between 9:30 and 11:30 this morning."

The morning passes, Mrs. Bateman feels worse, and the doctor has not called. She has carefully kept her phone line clear.

By 12:30, she decides to call again. "This is Mrs. Bateman again. I'm sorry to bother you, but when is the doctor going to call?"

"Oh, my, he's finished with office hours and is off for the afternoon. I gave him the message."

Mrs. Bateman had every right to feel betrayed and angry. She had called her doctor in good faith when she was ill and the call was not returned. Since he did not leave for an emergency, she felt he had no reason not to call her back. Her doctor will have to apologize and make a few phone calls on time to gain back her trust.

Occasionally, your doctor may not see the facts of your situation as they actually are. Perhaps you did not say anything to him; perhaps you didn't say enough. Perhaps you said it, but he didn't really hear you. Sometimes, a doctor loses his objectivity.

Jennifer's relationship with her doctor is in trouble:

"Good morning, Doctor."

"Good morning, Mary. Do I have any calls to return? Who is my first patient?"

"No calls yet, and your first patient is Jonas Lake. He has an infected hand. Oh, by the way, how is Jennifer?"

"Okay. When I saw her today, she told me all about Susie, her youngest. That little dickens won a first place at the State Fair for her sugar cookies, and that recipe was the one she got from my wife."

"You know, Doctor, that I really care about Jennifer. She's such a special person. I don't know if I should say anything, but. . . ."

"Say what?"

"Well, yesterday while you were gone, her husband stopped by for her prescription. He seemed so upset and preoccupied. Finally, he blurted out that Jennifer seems to be getting worse. He says that she cries at the drop of a hat, that her pain is worse than ever, and that her back hurts a lot."

"Really? How could I have missed anything? Jen and I have such a special relationship. I first saw her when she was only ten. Her mother brought her in with an awful case of poison ivy. We really hit it off then."

"I feel like I am butting in, Dr. Rollings, but maybe you are too close to Jennifer to assess her medical condition. Perhaps it's time to call in another doctor for a second opinion."

This situation should never have happened. Dr. Rollings was so taken with Jennifer as a person that he couldn't see Jennifer as a patient, too. In spite of, or because of his relationship with Jennifer and her family, he was blind to at least some of her symptoms.

Jennifer was at fault as well. She was guilty of not telling her doctor all he needed to know. She was inadvertently holding back some symptoms, not purposely perhaps, but simply because she had never had a situation such as chronic illness to deal with before. Perhaps she wanted to remain on her doctor's good side or conceal her noncompliance.

The doctor was only hearing what he wanted to hear, and Jennifer was only telling him what she thought he wanted to hear.

ADVOCATING FOR YOURSELF

Your job is to do everything in your power to help your doctor help you. Your doctor's job is to do everything he can to help you help yourself. This means you are going to have to become adept at asking questions and really listening to the answers.

Be reasonable, and use your common sense. Ask what you have a reason for asking. Very few doctors are going to ask patients whether they are having any problems beyond medicines, exercises, or other therapy. It is up to you to speak up.

It will take you a while to learn what to ask. These are good questions:

1. I'm having a lot of trouble sleeping. Do you have any suggestions to help me?
2. My feet are giving me so much trouble. Is that part of my illness? How should I handle the problem?
3. I can't tie my shoelaces or button my buttons. What can I do to help myself?
4. I have had some problems with dizziness in the last two weeks. Do you have any idea what might be causing it?
5. My hands hurt when I use my crutches. What can I do to stop that?
6. I know this sounds dumb, but I can't unscrew jar lids very often. Is there anything available which will help?

Not all your problems and concerns will be evident in the beginning of your illness. As your condition changes, your needs may change as well. Keep a running list of questions to ask your doctor. (You may be surprised how many you can cross out because they have just gone away!)

A journal or list of observations about your illness is a very useful tool, especially in the beginning of your condition, when you see the doctor infrequently, or when you start to notice a distinct change. Your list should include any changes in your condition and how you are reacting to a new medicine. Make it as specific as possible. How long did the pain last? Could you grip and hold a large bowl? How many steps could you take? Here is an example of a good list. Notice the attention paid to the sequence of events.

9/21/82: Noticing feelings of weakness in my arms and hands. Could not clench fist without pain.

9/23/82: Dropped and broke two glasses. Pain when I lift arm as high as shoulder. Heating pad for half hour helped.

9/25/82: Numbness in fingers of right hand (placed call to doctor; he set up an immediate appointment to see me).

Here's another example:

7/7/84: Dizziness several times today, seems unrelated.

7/10/84: Very frustrated because legs aren't very strong.

7/22/84: Forgot to take medicine to work, called doctor. He altered course of therapy for the day.

7/22/84: Very constipated—not a usual problem for me.

The items on your list may seem to be isolated incidents when they occur, but the doctor may be able to see a pattern or relationship soon enough to head off a problem. He should be told at each visit about any new problems. Notice 7/22/84 above. She knew she had a problem and called to find out how to handle it.

BE PREPARED WHEN YOU SEE OR TALK WITH YOUR DOCTOR

Now, before you rush down to your doctor with pages and pages of questions, stop and organize yourself.

You have to be sure you encourage your doctor's respect by calling or making an appointment only when necessary. Being prepared for your visits or phone calls to your doctor is an important way to show your active, thoughtful, and conscientious participation on your own health care team.

Alan Brown could have avoided this problematic exchange if he'd been better prepared for his appointment:

Dr. Bradley: "Good morning, Mr. Brown. How are you this beautiful day? I see you're in for your 6 month visit about your Parkinson's disease. Let me see you walk, please. (Dr. Bradley continues his examination.) Mr. Brown, I'm noticing a little more rigidity in your arms. I'd like you to see the physical therapist. She'll teach you some range-of-motion exercises which should be helpful for you. Let me know if any other problems arise. Get dressed now, and I'll be right back with the orders for the physical therapy."

Alan Brown: (Mr. Brown is dressed now and Dr. Bradley re-enters the room with the orders. As Mr. Brown is shaking Dr. Bradley's hand, he mentions:) "Say, do you think it's anything important if I can't sleep lying down? Lately I get too short of breath if I do."

Dr. Bradley now has a new, and probably important, symptom to work with. Mr. Brown has to undress again, and the doctor begins his examination again, this time for a different reason.

I have heard this kind of behavior described as a "door knob" problem because the patient literally has his or her hand on the door knob before the problem is mentioned.

You can prepare yourself for an office visit or phone call to your doctor by first asking yourself (and answering!) the following questions.

1. How long have I been feeling such-and-such a way?
2. What, exactly, are my symptoms?
3. Have I lost or gained any weight?
4. What do I do that causes pain or discomfort?
5. At what time of the day are my symptoms the worst?
6. Have I been running a fever? For how long? How high? At what times of the day?
7. Am I getting enough sleep?
8. Have I been under an unusual amount of stress?

You and your doctor will get much more out of your office visit or phone call if you follow this format. You're in control, so don't waste your time or the time of your doctor.

Let me stress another point. Don't hesitate to describe your emotional difficulties if and when they occur. If the doctor asks, "Well, how are you and your family adjusting?" and you respond with, "Just fine," or some other non-answer, your doctor can only assume that you mean what you say. In fact, you may be miserable trying to cope with a family that doesn't understand many problems you barely understand yourself. It's important to tell the truth. It's okay to reply, "My children and my wife are all acting as though I'm made of fine china, and I don't know how to handle the problem." Another example would be, "I don't know why I cry or get angry so easily now. I think I'm driving my family crazy. Does it have anything to do with my illness?"

Some people are reluctant to speak frankly because they are afraid of sounding like complainers. This is no time to be macho or a martyr. Doctors know that adjustment to a chronic illness can cause emotional stress and they expect to hear about it. Denying emotional difficulties can only harm your overall well-being. Try to be honest with yourself and your physician.

Let's look at examples of an office visit which reflects good preparation on the part of the patient:

Dr. Soristo: "Mrs. Fremsted, it's nice to see you again. How are you feeling?"

Mary Fremsted: "Actually, not very well, Doctor. I've taken the medicine for my angina exactly as you prescribed when I saw you two weeks ago, but the chest pain doesn't seem any better. What can we do now?"

Dr. Soristo: "I'm glad you've come back to see me. I'd still like to stick with this medication for a little longer, but I'll increase the dose slightly. This time, call me after a week if the medicine still isn't working and we'll see if we can't make you more comfortable. There are several other drugs we can try. I'll have my nurse do an electrocardiogram, and then I'll listen to your chest. Is anything else bothering you?"

Mary Fremsted: "No, Dr. Soristo, but I'll sure be glad when this chest pain gets better."

Dr. Soristo: (After examining Mrs. Fremsted) "Everything else seems fine. Now don't forget to call me in a week. Then we'll see how you are doing. Call me sooner if the pain changes or becomes more severe."

A visit such as this one encourages Dr. Soristo's respect for Mrs. Fremsted. It's just as obvious that she respects his time and takes care of her own health. They make a good team.

The need to be prepared applies equally to phone calls to your doctor. Here's an example of how *not* to make a call to your physician:

"Hello, Dr. Smith? I'm calling because my wife is having a problem. She says she feels just terrible."

—"Honey, the doctor wants to know what the problem is. Do you have a fever?"—

"She didn't take her temperature but she says she feels warm."

This type of call is very frustrating to the physician. In the first place, unless the patient is absolutely unable to come to the phone, he will want to speak to her directly, regardless of how poorly she is feeling. He needs to hear her voice to get a sense of the problem. Also, the doctor needs specific information, most of which can be anticipated. He shouldn't be forced to ask a time-consuming series of questions to determine for himself whether an actual emergency prompted her call.

Compare the last example with these:

"Hello, my name is Manuel Gonzales and I am Dr. Johnson's patient. I am 44 years old and have multiple sclerosis. My medicines are _____, _____, and _____. A few minutes ago when I got up to urinate, I couldn't pass any urine. I'm in severe pain with a full bladder. What should I do now?"

This description gets to the point. The physician has most of the information he needs to help this patient. With a few more questions, he can begin to take appropriate action.

"My name is Susan Swanson and I am Dr. Scanlon's patient. I am 65 years old, I have rheumatoid arthritis and am taking _____, _____, _____, and _____. About an hour ago, my knee started hurting more than usual, and became so painful that it kept me awake. Now I have a fever of over 103 degrees and my entire knee is red and swollen. What do you recommend?"

Susan has helped herself by presenting a concise, specific situation. The doctor may continue to ask questions, but it sounds as if Susan is ready with the answers!

These people were prepared. They didn't waste time explaining symptoms which were irrelevant to the condition that prompted the phone call. Most doctors appreciate this. They will soon learn they can trust you to call only when it's really necessary. In return, you will consistently get their full cooperation.

To help yourself be prepared, think ahead. Most of the questions you will be asked can be anticipated and planned for. Keep a list of information posted near the phone where both you and your family can find it easily. Your list should include:

1. Name and current symptoms of your chronic illness (i.e., "I have systemic lupus erythematosus. I suffer from flares with fever, joint pain, and exhaustion.").
2. The name of your physician and how to reach him. Include all his phone numbers.
3. Which hospital you should be taken to in case of emergency.
4. Complete health insurance information, including the company name, policy numbers, and phone numbers.
5. The names of all medicines you are currently taking. State exact dosages and the number of times you take them each day.
6. A complete, up-to-date list of allergies and other drug sensitivities.
7. Your pharmacy phone number, and the phone number of an alternate if the first one is closed.
8. Your address. Include a cross street for emergency vehicles. Your address is important because a friend or neighbor may need to place an emergency call for you and not know your address off hand.
9. The name and phone number (home and work) of a trusted person other than a relative.

Being able to communicate calmly and accurately so your doctor really understands your situation allows you to be an effective promoter of your own health. *No one but you knows what your concerns are. If you don't impart them clearly to your doctor, no one but you will ever know.*

CHANGING DOCTORS

The possibility exists in all long-term relationships that things won't work out between the two people involved. Doctors and their patients are no exception. Before deciding to change doctors, however, do everything possible to mend the relationship. Starting over with a new doctor takes time and effort; you should first try to make the most of your investment with your present physician.

Begin by taking a close look at your reasons for wanting a change. Do you have a good reason? Some people switch doctors simply to avoid facing a frightening diagnosis or difficult treatment plan. Switching doctors is not easy and can interrupt the continuity of care required to treat a chronic illness.

If, after careful thought, you conclude that your doctor is not meeting his obligations to you, grant him the courtesy of a frank discussion. Sit down with him and discuss your feelings honestly. You might discover that your doctor has absolutely no idea you are dissatisfied. Most doctors genuinely care about their patients and are willing to try to meet any reasonable expectations.

In the real world, however, there are unavoidable times when two well-meaning people simply can't agree. If you and your doctor cannot come to terms about your treatment, use deliberation and care to make a change. Try to avoid anger and bad feelings toward your former doctor. Finally, make sure to have all your records transferred—you want to be certain that your new doctor fully understands your medical situation.

TO MY DOCTOR

I am not just a chart number
I am not "what's his name"
I'm a living, loving person
With feelings and a brain.

I'll try to answer honestly
And expect the same from you.
Together we will make a team
*And we **will** pull me through.*

——*Sefra Pitzele, 1984*

YOUR PHARMACIST

Your pharmacist can and should be a member of your health care team. Choose one pharmacy you can use conveniently and regularly. Most pharmacies now keep a drug profile on each patient. This is a list with all the known drugs that patient is currently taking as well as medicine allergies. More than once I have heard stories about pharmacists preventing possible dangerous drug interactions by recognizing the conflict and calling it to the attention of the patient or the doctor.

Contrary to what you may believe, pharmacists do more than just count pills. They are a valuable resource about over-the-counter remedies, and often are asked for help in choosing the appropriate non-prescription medicine for their customers. After a time, your pharmacist will recognize you, ask how you are doing, and become a valuable part of your health care team.

YOUR HOSPITAL TEAM

At one time or another, most of us will spend some time in the hospital. Consequently, your health care team will include members of the hospital staff: aides, lab technicians, administrative personnel, therapists and, most important of all, nurses.

The T.V. portrayal of these dedicated angels of mercy as all-knowing and always supportive is a myth. Just like doctors, they are individual people who require your understanding and cooperation. The orientation of the hospital organization is toward acute care, so when you check in, you're going to have to work at building good relationships. A little insight may prepare you to receive treatment that is somewhat different from what you might expect.

While most health care professionals are very conscientious, caring individuals, you may occasionally encounter some negative comments from some hospital personnel. The admissions clerk might greet you with, "Oh, are you back again? You don't look too bad. What's going on?" You might sense that the floor nurse is sending up a silent prayer *not* to be assigned to your case, again. Like it or not, you and the hospital staff have to work together. If you are ever to meet your health care needs, you must suppress any feelings of self-pity or resentment, and try to understand why many hospital professionals dislike treating chronically ill people.

First of all, the very word *chronic* carries negative connotations. Who hasn't heard of the chronic complainer, the chronic sinus infection, or the chronically depressed person? Our diagnosis projects a poor image from the start.

The lack of cooperation shown by some chronically ill patients during administrative procedures has further reinforced the stereotypes held by many hospital staff people. It is understandable, but not excusable, that we would be tempted to resent or respond flippantly to routine administrative questions. We're tired and in pain and the last thing we need is an interrogation from a nurse or desk clerk.

What does it matter, we wonder, whether we have dentures, more than $5.00 in our pocket, or previous surgery? After all, a lot of this information is in our hospital records, or we have already answered similar questions in the emergency room if we were admitted there.

This kind of situation is just as frustrating for the nurse or admitting desk clerk. Questions that seem trivial or repetitive to us are critical to the admissions process. The staff can't rely on your records because it often takes an hour or more to get them from the records room. The information from the emergency room is not always reliable—in the stress and pain of an emergency room situation, we don't always think straight and may inadvertently answer a question incompletely or incorrectly.

Probably the most infuriating reply a patient can make is, "My doctor knows all those answers." So what? Maybe he does remember every detail of every case; it still is a poor use of everyone's time to interview the doctor instead of you! Remember, the staff carries out the doctor's orders, and they can't do so properly until all the administrative details have been addressed. The modern hospital runs on good information, and you have to help them help you. Take a deep breath, answer their questions clearly, and get started on the right foot.

An experienced nurse I spoke with suggested that chronically ill patients should keep a small, typed sheet of all pertinent information in their wallet or purse, and simply give it to the people who need the information. The information on this sheet might include medical condition, medications, the nature and dates of past surgeries, and any allergies and sensitivities. I only wish I had heard this outstanding idea earlier! It saves everyone time and trouble, and suggests that you are a well-organized person who respects the staff's need for information.

The frustrations of treating chronic illness can confuse and aggravate the nursing staff. We just aren't like other patients. For one thing, we frequently don't look sick. Nor are our symptoms as dramatic as those of acutely ill patients. We're also unpredictable. With some illnesses, symptoms can change abruptly. We also come across as demanding because we understand our bodies and our illnesses better than most of the staff, and we're quick to notice errors or omissions in our medication. Because of the quirks of chronic illness, some nurses might feel that we're malingering and complaining.

Another aspect of our care that many nurses find frustrating is the fact that we do not exhibit signs of pain that are readily identifiable. Chronically ill patients frequently do not display the symptoms which the hospital staff has been trained to associate with pain, such as agitation, pallor, increased pulse, or moaning. Many of us have developed an ability to tolerate the intrusion of severe pain, often daily. We may also have learned techniques like relaxation therapy or self-hypnosis to control our pain. Consequently, nurses and other members of the hospital staff may not be as inclined to help us as they would a patient who displays more typical pain symptoms.

This is a credibility problem. The hospital staff is trained to objectively observe certain symptoms before administering pain medication. They are very careful about this because they risk creating or reinforcing a substance abuse problem. What do we do? Allow ourselves to show the pain we've worked so hard to control? Let the pain progress and get out of hand so we exhibit normal symptoms? Or should we forget all about stoicism in a hospital setting and let ourselves fall apart just to get noticed?

The appropriate course lies somewhere between pretending we don't hurt and letting go completely. We shouldn't have to give up the lessons of self-control to get attention, but we can still allow ourselves to relinquish control to our health care team. Ask yourself: What do I need to do or say to feel better faster?

I encountered this situation when I was recently hospitalized for a lupus flare. Although I looked fairly normal, there were times when I could no longer control the pain and I needed medication. Although the nurses always brought it willingly enough, I sensed some skepticism on their part. Since I can manage pain fairly well, they didn't see the type of behavior that would have convinced them I was really hurting.

That experience convinced me that negative, skeptical attitudes toward chronic illness don't go away until we, as patients, take the initiative to communicate more.

Ever since, I speak to each nurse assigned to my care. I explain what my pain is like and what pain control techniques I have learned to use. I emphasize that I can only control my pain up to a certain point; beyond that point, I really do need their help, even though it might not be apparent. I hope that by communicating honestly with the hospital staff before a problem develops, we can establish the mutual respect and understanding so necessary to good team-work and good health care.

Here are some other suggestions which can strengthen your relationships with your hospital health care team:

1. No matter how much insensitivity or lack of understanding you encounter, do not allow yourself the luxury of impatience or self-pity. Patients are so named because we're suppose to be patient! You may find it difficult to be reasonable all the time, but remember that being a demanding, negative patient reinforces an unfair stereotype of yourself and other people with chronic illness.

2. If you are dissatisfied with a staff member's performance, you should first consider overlooking it. Like doctors, nurses and other members of the hospital staff are human; they can make mistakes and have off days. However, if the quality of health care has seriously suffered from an unsatisfactory performance, or you are concerned about a pattern of behavior that looks like a problem waiting to happen, speak up loud and clear. Write or speak to that person's supervisor or to the patient advocate (if your hospital has such a person). The tone of your communication should be calm, factual, and fair. Temper tantrums and idle threats never resolve anything.

3. Don't overlook the positive! If a hospital staff member has taken extra time to make you comfortable or has come up with especially helpful suggestions for your treatment, be sure to praise him or her. Likewise, let the person's supervisor know. We all want and need positive recognition.

Your doctor can be a strong ally in your efforts to build cooperation and understanding with the hospital staff. Some doctors try to place chronically ill hospital patients on certain floors or in areas better suited to care for them. A doctor can also call a formal or an impromptu *care conference* to discuss your situation. A care conference can involve just the immediate staff, or also include the psychologist, social worker, dietician, and others who are contributing to your care effort.

During the care conference, the physician explains you have again been admitted to the hospital, what he hopes to achieve, and how the nursing staff and others can help. The staff can air their concerns and ideas as well. This method of conferencing reinforces the sense of teamwork to "share the care." The nurses, in particular, have a better understanding of how they can best attend to your needs. With more information and a better perspective, they can make more knowledgeable observations about your response to the treatment program.

Let me emphasize once again that you must maintain a good, honest relationship with your extended health care team. They are as important as your doctor because they deliver the care prescribed. You can depend on them, but it is up to you to be certain that you are a participant in your health care, not just a recipient. Your job as a patient is to do everything in your power to help them help you. Mutual respect and cooperation will help you, your doctor, and the hospital staff meet your common goal: Keeping you as healthy and pain-free as possible.

REGAINING INDEPENDENCE

Slowly, with the help of your doctor and your health care team, you will begin to regain your independence. As you gain more experience with your condition, your self-confidence will return.

Learning to depend upon your own judgment again is a tricky maneuver when you have a chronic illness. Regrettably, you may no sooner learn to stand on your own two feet again when another flare occurs and you are once again dependent on your physician. You are, and will always be, the unwilling victim of your medical condition.

Imagine your chronic illness or medical condition as a leash. As you struggle to get off the leash, a flare of your illness may occur and once again you are jerked or pulled back to a state of dependency.

As you become used to the physical changes that occur, as you become used to the discomfort and inconvenience, and as you become used to the persistence of chronic illness symptoms, you will find your need for your doctor and your health care team diminishing. This, too, is normal.

Several months after your diagnosis, if you find yourself as dependent as you were in the beginning of your illness, it is time to evaluate why. Do you have friends or family with whom you can talk? Have you reached out into your community for support? Are you taking the time to nourish your social and emotional needs?

Carefully evaluate why you are making each phone call. It is *not* normal to continue to need the physician the way you did when your condition was first diagnosed.

Evaluate your behavior. Is your dependence on your physician too important to you? Are you reluctant to trust yourself? Are you having trouble accepting responsibility for your comfort and health? Do you need to rethink your relationship with your doctor? Try to answer these questions for yourself, and if you feel you have become too dependent, make some positive moves to gain back your independence.

DELICATE SCAFFOLD

Framework, network, listening post
Doctor, family, nurse, and me.
Building strength from a delicate scaffold
Maintaining trust and sanity.

Like building a home, our trust will grow
Piece by honest piece.
Until we're done and we can see
We've made a new structure to hold up me.

——SEFRA PITZELE, 1984

MAKING DAILY CHOICES

With a chronic illness or medical condition, each day is going to be a special challenge. After you have had the illness for a while, you will find that you will know better what is important and what is not. You will learn to judge for yourself whether to call the doctor or try to solve the problem alone.

Your days will be full of choices that may involve your health care team. Your life will once again develop meaningful patterns, and your optimism and self-confidence will return. There is no reason to slow down the process of acceptance and adaptation by being a poor patient.

Remember to be a participant in your health care, not just a recipient—You're a strong player on your own wellness team. Your job as a patient is to do everything in your power to help your health care team help you. Relationships based on mutual respect and cooperation permit your doctor, nurses, and the other professionals on your team to meet your common goal: Keeping you healthy and painfree.

THE CIRCLE OF STRESS, ILLNESS, AND PAIN

Pain will come and go throughout your life. Some of it will be caused by your chronic medical condition, and some will be caused by other stressful circumstances. Since you know that there may often be some pain, you have to learn to allow the pain to become a part of your life, but not *all* of your life. You can control your pain. Do not let pain control your life.

Rows and rows of pharmacy shelves are devoted to pain-relievers. Pain is a *very* prevalent problem, even among people who do not have a chronic problem with their health. In fact, an amazing one billion dollars a year is spent just on over-the-counter pain remedies. Sales of prescription drugs are similarly high. Codeine, for example, has annual sales in excess of $400 million dollars!

Without a chronic illness in the picture, the average American loses at least two weeks of productivity each year due to pain. When we add the pain-related productivity loss due to a chronic medical condition, we have a much more serious problem. Anyone who lives in constant pain knows that life can, indeed, become almost unbearable.

There are essentially two types of pain, acute and chronic. By its very nature, acute pain demands and receives immediate attention. Regardless of the cause, it is very likely that the physician will either hospitalize the patient who has acute pain or send him home with a specific regimen to follow until the severity of the pain diminishes. Chronic pain is less understood.

It takes some time to adjust to chronic pain. Pain can be pervasive and can intrude upon your whole being until you begin to think that there is nothing left in your life but coping with the pain.

THE CIRCLE OF STRESS, ILLNESS, AND PAIN

For everyone, and especially for those with a chronic medical condition, pain and stress are intertwined. Pain is your body's reaction to stress-inducing events, activities, or conditions. These mental or physical "stressors" can cause a short-term or long-term aggravation of your chronic condition, and in turn cause pain. The circle below illustrates this relationship:

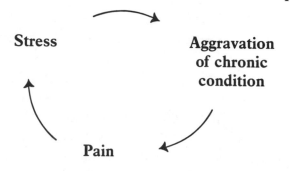

Stress

Aggravation of chronic condition

Pain

All by itself, your chronic illness causes stress when it strains your body, mind, or spirit. When you add all the other stressful events which occur in your daily life, you should realize that the effects of this new norm will be tougher to handle.

WHAT IS STRESS?

Before chronic illness entered our lives, most of us perceived stress as a negative event occurring in an isolated fashion. "The good old days" were those days when the worst strains on you were simpler and less frequent: Changing jobs, misplacing your house keys, or being called away from work because your child needed stitches. Each incident was isolated. After it was dealt with, it was over.

When you have a chronic illness, however, stress and its effects are not isolated incidents. Stress, chronic illness, and pain are all intertwined. You can significantly improve your quality of life by learning to recognize and cope more effectively with the stress you can control.

The sources of stress can be either physical or emotional, and each can dramatically affect your health and the amount of pain you have. The most obvious examples of physical stress come from your daily activities.

Lifting groceries and carrying them upstairs, doing yard work, or hiking across a huge suburban parking lot are examples of common physical stressors. These are not major activities when you're in good health, but they take on a different significance when you have a chronic medical condition.

You may also have a physical reaction to something you perceive as an acute threat. Your body responds totally automatically with what is known as the "fight or flight" reaction.

> Harvey was taking a short walk around his block after work, a habit he'd gotten into after his doctor told him he should exercise to improve the muscle tone in his legs. He was learning to adjust to the fact that his hiking days were over, and even though the walk seemed to take a little longer each day, he enjoyed the private time to relax and collect his thoughts before joining his family for dinner.
>
> As he rounded the corner at the back of the apartment building, he heard a sharp "crack" in the bushes a few yards away. A husky teenage boy dashed out, straight at him. Harvey turned sideways, hoping to blunt the attack, but realized instantly that he was no match. He froze, and his once strong legs tensed—but they were worthless now.
>
> The young man veered to the left and raced past Harvey. Then a teenage girl burst out of the same place, heading in the opposite direction.
>
> "Gosh," Harvey gasped, starting to breathe again. "It was only two teenagers necking behind the building." But his heart was still beating wildly, and his legs were shaking as he walked home.

During the "fight or flight" reaction, your body readies itself to handle the threat:

■ Your heart beats faster.

■ Adrenaline surges through your bloodstream, often causing a part of your body to shake uncontrollably.

- Muscles tense.
- You begin to sweat.
- Your digestive system slows down.

All these physical stresses cut into your already depleted stores of energy, and can drain your resistance even further.

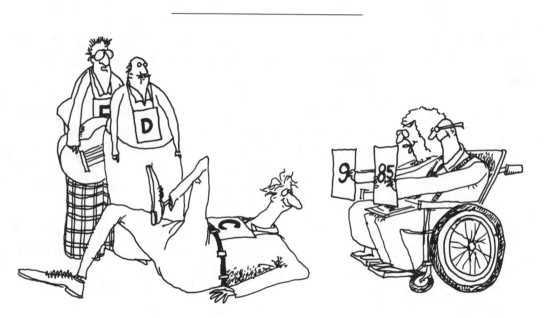

Some people take the art of falling very seriously.

Perhaps even more significant to your health is the effect of *emotional stress*. We have experienced emotional stress all our lives. Remember some of the simple emotional stressors you had as a child? If only we could go back to the days of crying because the barber cut off too much hair, or moping by the phone for a Saturday night date!

As an adult with a chronic condition, however, all the normal emotional stresses of living in our fast-paced, computerized, twentieth-century world are magnified. Waiting in a long line at the supermarket becomes impossible.

Tiredness becomes uncontrollable fatigue, and pain, tolerated all day, seems to explode in the evening. Minor problems, such as being unable to open a medicine bottle, can make you burst into tears. Every task, even opening a door, throws another roadblock in your way.

Your body "reads" the signals it's getting. Unfortunately, it can't tell whether the exhaustion is from the emotional stress of a vacation or family problem, or a reaction to the physical stress of doing too much yard work. These factors, which all cause stress, often cause pain as well.

HOW STRESS AFFECTS YOUR HEALTH

In 1967, two psychiatrists published the following chart that lists stress-inducing events felt by adults. Each stressor is rated according to its level of impact. I have seen this chart many times, but it wasn't until I developed a chronic illness that I really began to pay attention to it. Read the list of events listed in the left column, and make a check mark by each that has occurred in your life in the last year.

EVENT	SCALE OF IMPACT
Death of spouse	100
Divorce	73
Marital separation	65
Jail term	63
Death of close family member	63
Personal injury or illness	53
Marriage	50
Fired at work	47
Marital reconciliation	45
Retirement	45
Change in health of family member	44
Pregnancy	40
Sex difficulties	39
Gain of new family member	39
Business readjustment	39
Change in financial state	38
Death of close friend	37

Change to different line of work 36
Change in number of arguments with spouse................35
Mortgage or loan for major purchase (home, etc.)...........31
Foreclosure of mortgage or loan........................30
Change in responsibilities at work.........................29
Son or daughter leaving home 29
Trouble with in-laws...............................29
Outstanding personal achievement 28
Wife begins or stops work 26
Begin or end school.............................26
Change in living conditions........................25
Revision of personal habits.........................24
Trouble with boss 23
Change in work hours or conditions 20
Change in residence............................20
Change in schools..............................20
Change in recreation 19
Change in church activities........................19
Change in social activities.........................18
Mortgage or loan for lesser purchase (car, T.V., etc.) 17
Change in sleeping habits 16
Change in number of family get-togethers 15
Change in eating habits.........................15
Vacation 13
Christmas 12
Minor violation of the law............................11

"The Social Readjustment Rating Scale" was developed by Thomas H. Holmes, M.D., and Richard H. Rahe, M.D., and first appeared in the Journal of Psychosomatic Research, Vol. II, p. 216, in 1967. It is reprinted with the permission of Microform International Marketing Corporation, exclusive copyright licensee of Pergamon Press Journal back files.

Now add the scores of the events you checked off. A score of 150 indicates that you have about a fifty-fifty possibility of developing a stress-related health change. If your score totals more than 300, your chance for a significant health change escalates to about 90%.

As you went through the chart, did you notice how many events may now affect you solely because you have a chronic medical condition? As much as I hate to admit it, there are many items here that are pertinent to each of us.

It is, for example, unfortunate but true that people who have chronic illnesses tend to get divorced or separated more than other groups in the general population. Additionally, you may experience events such as change in health of a family member, sex difficulties, change in work responsibilities, and even change in sleeping habits. It doesn't take too long to figure out that those of us who have a chronic medical condition are at very high risk on this stress scale.

Notice also that stress is not only caused by negative events. A much-desired marriage or birth of a child may be a very positive event—but each causes a great deal of emotional stress that may have significant impact on those with a chronic condition.

Everyone is affected at one time or another by life changes such as these. When many changes occur over a short period of time, stress increases. The importance of this chart is that it can help identify those people who are more prone to the onset of physical illness or the painful aggravation of a chronic condition. The chart does not predict illness, but it can help make you more aware if you are at greater risk.

WHAT YOU CAN DO TO INTERRUPT THE CIRCLE

The first step in interrupting the circle of stress, illness, and pain is to recognize that your health, and the amount of pain you have, are affected by stress.

Remember that stress can be either physical or emotional, and has different levels of impact. Major stress can be caused by the events listed in the previous chart, and minor physical and emotional stresses can result just from coping with daily problems.

One of the most powerful tools you can use to combat the effects of stress on your general health and your chronic illness is to change the pattern of stress. Try the following sequence of actions:

1. *Recognize* that stress plays a part in your life.
2. *Evaluate* why you have stress.
3. *Act* on your plan.
4. *Plan* positive life-style changes to reduce stress.
5. *Reap* the benefits of change.

Once you have recognized stress and decided to lessen it, here are some suggestions that may be helpful:

- Set realistic goals for yourself, both long-term and short-term.

- Structure your day so that you are in control of your time and activities.

- Get plenty of sleep.

- Share your thoughts, concerns, and problems with someone else. Internalizing your stress can make you physically ill.

- If possible, take a break away from the source of your stress.

- Drink and eat in moderation. Try to be as close as possible to your optimum weight.

- Monitor drug and substance use, including caffeine and nicotine.

- Make stress reduction a part of your everyday life.

Also, try to keep busy. If you are concentrating on something else, you will think less about being in pain. No one can make stress go away entirely, but we can keep it from accelerating the cycle of stress, illness, and pain.

If your pain is very serious, your physician may recommend a pain clinic. One of the first goals of a pain clinic is to stop existing pain from causing more pain. A pain clinic is usually a multi-disciplinary approach to harnessing pain, and is often found under one roof. For example, a low-back clinic may include a doctor, nurse, therapists, therapy equipment, a therapeutic swimming pool, and X-ray facilities.

In addition, exercise, biofeedback, imagery, or hypnotism may be taught as methods of controlling pain. It is up to the doctors and therapists to identify the most appropriate pain-remedy techniques for each patient.

Regardless of which you find most effective for you, your goal must be to *interrupt the circle of stress, illness, and pain.* Remember, you *can* do many things to control your pain. Keep working at it until you succeed. Don't let pain control your life.

Community: Most communities offer a variety of assistance and support services to local residents. Of particular significance are the many different coping and support groups available.

Sometimes the need for a coping group comes suddenly, and we find ourselves in the group whether we intended to be there or not. This type of group has as its focus the need to rehabilitate. In a setting like this, patients with a common medical problem can learn to adjust to their new medical situations by spending time with others with medical problems. For example, with a heart attack, daily classes may be mandatory for the couple during the recovery period. Rehabilitative support groups teach us about our medical situation, help with personal and family emotional needs, and send us on our way better prepared to live with our problem.

At other times, we may find ourselves in a support group for even more unexpected and tragic reasons, such as suffering the loss of a child to sudden infant death syndrome or the death of a loved one in an auto accident. These support groups are for people who have acute emotional needs and people participate as long as they need the support. Fortunately, most hospitals and physician's offices can help make immediate contact with this kind of group.

With chronic illness support groups, the situation is quite different. Sometimes we don't even perceive our need for a support group, at least not until several weeks or even months past the time of initial caring and close support from our family and friends. Now the need to learn to cope takes on a recognizable form in our mind, and may become a need to talk to other people who will understand what we face each day.

All of us who have a chronic illness have learned by now that even our own family members don't want or need to hear the mundane daily litany about our illness or what our day was like emotionally and physically. It is a boring thing to come home to, in either illness or in good health, and tends to make the home more like a hospital. None of us wants to hear every detail of anyone's life. Family members will, of course, still rise to the challenge when our days are very bad. However, generally within six months of the diagnosis or the first very bad episode, they expect we'll have some pain, discomfort, and inconveniences. They expect us to accept that as the new norm, too.

For many of us, this is the time that the absolute aloneness of our situation finally hits home. We commonly feel an overwhelming desire to talk with other people who share our condition.

Alcoholics Anonymous is an excellent example of a chronic illness support group. There is always strength in numbers, and an alcoholic has a far better chance of not drinking again if he can maintain a constant source of support. There are now similar groups for drug users, gamblers, dieters, physical abusers, and many more.

Chronic illness support groups typically meet once a month or once every other month, depending on the needs of the members. Since the need is on-going, support is needed on a continuing basis. The groups are always there, and we can choose whether we need to go or not. You may be able to go to a larger meeting in your city that is sponsored by the Arthritis Foundation, for example. The larger meetings usually have a speaker or a theme, such as exercise, how to make your work situation easier, or medicinal therapy. Question and answer sessions are common. From these larger meetings you may find out about smaller coping groups in your neighborhood.

If the group you begin attending is sponsored by an illness-oriented organization such as lupus, arthritis, or the Heart Foundation, one of the main goals of the group will be to keep you well educated on your illness and any new treatments. Many groups encourage family members to attend with you. But many spouses have all they can do to handle your chronic illness at home, and may be reluctant to become even more involved. Don't let your spouse's feelings in this case affect your decision of whether or not to attend, however. Your meeting time may be an opportunity for your spouse to have his or her private time, and he or she is entitled to that. Participate in a meaningful support group as often and as much as you feel is of benefit to you.

Imagine this scene:

There is a support group meeting and the husband is angry and resentful and doesn't want to go along.
The wife really wants him to go, mostly for emotional support, as she has not been to a meeting and is apprehensive about going alone.

SUPPORT GROUP

Tiny islands of people, two or three to a group
sitting
apart
from the others.
Wondering if they were dragged to this meeting too.

Only a few really wanted to attend.
The rest are captive . . . forced by husbands, wives, lovers, or friends.
Yanked from their own private hell—no one wants to share—

AND I WON'T EITHER!

Privately I say, "What a waste of time. I could be at home, watching the Monday night football game."

Chairs and people turn now, the speaker begins and starts to make some sense.

All right, I'll stay to see what he has to say.
Now can we go? Questions and answers? And coffee and cake?
What the hell. We're here anyway, what difference does it make?

That man over there is sharing some thoughts from deep within his soul.
And he hurts too.

But I'm a private person—sharing's not my goal.

Shake hands, leave, drive home, and finally say,
"I admit I was relieved to hear other people tell how they hate their lives and what's happened to them too.

I admit it—I learned, but I won't go back again. I hated being there.
I'll support you at home. You'll have to go to these alone."

——Sefra Pitzele, 1983

You may also be able to get help from a local *information and referral line.* If your city maintains such a service, you will usually find it listed under Human Services in the Yellow Pages. If you need help immediately and can't find the number, call your directory assistance operator. This information and referral service, sometimes called a Help Line or First Call for Help, will direct you to the appropriate agency for your specific problem.

In order to acquire a *handicapped parking permit*, you will have to call your city offices and find out which department administers the permits. Most applications require both you and your doctor to complete the form. Your handicapped permit will be temporary or permanent, depending upon the reason for obtaining it. Take care of it and don't lend it to anyone. Display it when you park according to your city's requirements.

Dealing with any assistance office: When dealing with any assistance office, it is wise to do the following:

1. Keep a list of frequently called phone numbers.
2. Call ahead and ask as many questions as you can by phone.
3. Ask to whom you are speaking.
4. Take notes, mark the date, and be sure you understand the answer. If not, ask for clarification. You may be able to save yourself a tiring trip.
5. Try not to call on days after legal holidays, Mondays, or on the first day of the month. These are the busiest days.
6. Note what hours the office is open.

Other helpful suggestions:

1. Beauty and barber schools are often willing to give free or inexpensive haircuts.
2. Congregate dining programs are available in many areas. The food is hot, good, nutritious, and nominally priced.
3. Bakeries, dairies, and produce companies often sell their day-old products at greatly reduced prices.
4. Grocery stores, especially on Monday mornings, have carts of produce, baked goods, and breads at very low prices.
5. Agencies such as Goodwill and church-sponsored stores sell clothing and household goods at low prices. Do not hesitate to take advantage of these facilities.

COMMENTS ON DEPRESSION:

"I've tried, but I'm still so sad..."

Why is a discussion of depression important to sufferers of chronic illness?

In general, those of us who have chronic, restrictive medical conditions are at higher risk for stress-related illnesses. In addition to all the normal pressures of life, we have the added burden of dealing with a medical problem which will never go away. Many of you will understand what I mean when I say that each day is full of its own set of battles.

Each day, we struggle to maintain our precarious emotional and physical balancing act. All day we weigh the pros and cons of which activities to perform and how much emotional and physical energy they merit. When something happens to disturb this equilibrium and we can no longer handle the stress, a loss of control in the form of depression may occur.

The depression I am referring to is more than the sadness associated with grieving. Clinical depression is usually prolonged and dysfunctional. It is important to recognize it early so that professional help can be sought. Since most of us are not routinely seeing a psychologist who would recognize the symptoms, we have to pay close attention to our own thoughts and feelings.

SADNESS IS NORMAL

Clinical or chronic depression may begin as a normal reaction to a saddening event. Feelings of sadness generally subside after several days or a few weeks as a part of the grieving process.

When feelings of grieving or sadness do not subside after a reasonable period of time, it may signal the onset of depression. Depression is a chronic disorder of a person's feelings. It is called an "affective disorder," and is the most common of these disorders. Affect, as it is used here, means how a person relates to himself and to his environment. The feelings experienced in this change of emotion often affect even physical movement.

> **"When you are feeling blue, go somewhere and watch children at play."**
>
> ——SEFRA PITZELE

Who you are, where you work, how you live, what color or religion you are, how tall or short you are, whether you are fat or thin or male or female are all unimportant. *No one* is exempt from depression.

When persistent feelings of gloom and loss of well-being do not diminish over time, and the feelings seem disproportionately overwhelming for the problem, it is time to speak to your physician about seeking further help.

It is generally believed that depression is largely caused by stress. Stress is often caused by emotional pressures. Depression, for some, is a reaction to loss of power or control over our own lives.

To a person already suffering from a restrictive chronic illness, depression compounds the problem. Depression can "turn your motor off" and cause you to stop fighting for a higher quality of life. One depression thought can lead to another, and before you know it, you have let go of your self-esteem and will power. Soon, you don't care about anything. The longer this dysfunctional attitude and behavior lasts, the harder it becomes to fight back. Somehow, the downward slide must be stopped.

Many events can trigger a bout with depression. Here are a few examples:

1. A person close to you dies.
2. You suffer a major disappointment at your job.
3. A strongly held belief is threatened or shattered (such as a religious or political conviction).

4. You fail at a relationship that is very important to you, such as marriage, a love affair, or a business relationship.
5. You relocate and suddenly lack close friends.
6. You assume a new and very stressful job.
7. You are diagnosed as having a chronic illness.

"Every person must believe in something. Try believing in yourself for a change!"

——SEFRA PITZELE

TYPES OF DEPRESSION

There are two basic categories of depression:

1. *Endogenous* depression, caused primarily by forces within the body.
2. *Exogenous* depression, caused primarily by forces outside of the body.

Endogenous depression might occur when the body lacks a vital mineral or hormone needed to maintain internal biological balance. Endogenous depression could be caused by illness as well.

Violet knew she was depressed. She couldn't explain why, but she knew it all the same. Something wasn't right. She was gaining weight, and it didn't seem that she had eaten that much extra food. Before Violet realized what was happening, she had gained 45 pounds.

She was also so gosh-darn exhausted all the time. It seemed to Violet that she barely had the strength to get out of bed in the morning and go to work.

Her physical problems were affecting her emotionally, as well, causing her to feel sad and discouraged all the time. No matter what she tried, she couldn't seem to shake it.

Finally, mostly because of the extreme fatigue, Violet made an appointment to see her family doctor. He examined her and did a blood test.

A few days later the doctor called Violet to report, "Your blood test shows that you are not producing nearly enough thyroid. I'll call your pharmacy right away to get you on some thyroid medicine. You should start to feel better within a few weeks."

Much to Violet's delight, she did begin to feel better. She began to lose the weight she had gained and her old peppiness returned. There *was* a problem, her body gave her a signal, and she was able to correct the problem.

Exogenous depression, on the other hand, is usually caused by events outside of the body. Events such as the loss of a loved one, loss of a job, loss of material possessions, or the loss of good health can trigger depression. For a person suffering from depression, the grieving time is disproportionate to the loss. For example:

Paul was involved in a terrible automobile accident. Paul was not injured, but his car was hit from behind and crashed into the car ahead of him, killing a small boy who was in the car.

The policeman who arrived at the scene of the accident realized that the icy road conditions were the main cause of the accident. After dispatching the ambulances to the hospital, the policeman realized that Paul was becoming increasingly distraught.

The policeman tried to calm Paul. "It's not your fault, Mister. You couldn't avoid the accident. You got hit from behind, remember?"

Paul was inconsolable. "He was just about the age of my son. Oh, my God, what have I done? I'll never forgive myself. Never."

The policeman finally called for another ambulance and sent Paul to the emergency room. Paul was admitted to the psychiatric ward. He needed several days of intensive counseling and support before his mental state improved to the point where he could be released.

Depression is a form of mental illness, and it is just as real as influenza or chicken-pox. Attempts to humor or cheer up the person who is mentally ill are as fruitless as trying to talk a person out of appendicitis.

RECOGNIZING THE NEED FOR HELP

Recognizing the need for help is much easier said than done.

Few people would deny that they feel episodes of the blues. The blues may vary from sadness after a movie that lingers for several hours to lamenting the end of a love affair. Even children get the blues.

---

66 If you are alone and finances permit, get a pet. Animals love you no matter what happens. 99

——SEFRA PITZELE

When sad feelings don't go away after what seems to be an appropriate period of time, or they seem to get worse, it is time to ask for help.

Often a person will not ask for help with depression because of a fear of being labeled mentally ill or emotionally "weak." This is an understandable concern, but would you deny yourself surgery to repair a broken leg? Why, then, would a person deny himself professional assistance for depression? Depression is just as real as a broken leg.

Jack had a stroke which left him with some impaired ability. A few months later, he had a severe heart attack. Jack's friends soon noticed that he hardly ever went to bed at a routine time, and when he did, he rarely slept more than two hours. He couldn't seem to concentrate, especially during their weekly poker games!

Jack had also spoken a few times of "ending it all, so I'm not a burden to anyone anymore." And, against his doctor's orders, he had gained 25 pounds in three months.

Jack's friends held an impromptu conference after one of the poker games. They enlisted Jack's brother, Arnie, to call Jack's doctor and express their concern. Immediately after Arnie's call, Jack's doctor placed a call to Jack and told him of his friends' concerns. He said that it sounded as though Jack might be depressed, and he would like to see Jack soon.

Jack was furious and refused to make a special appointment. "I'm not depressed—just mad about that lousy heart attack." Nevertheless, depression continued to wear on Jack, despite his protests to the contrary.

Jack didn't receive help until shortly thereafter when he had an acute attack of gout. Since Jack could hardly walk, there was no way to avoid a confrontation with the doctor. The doctor, alert now to the problem, was able to discuss depression and its treatment with Jack.

When the symptoms of depression interfere with a person's life and keep him from living as he has been accustomed, the time has come to get professional help. The obvious way to get help is to consult your regular physician. He may begin treatment or refer you to a psychiatrist or psychologist. There are also mental health centers in most cities that accept self-referrals.

As a person's life situation changes, so can a person's mental health. Depression can occur over and over again. Most of us are acquainted with someone who has had post-partum depression after the birth of a child.

Bryan and Maria had their first child, a beautiful six-pound baby boy. They were both ecstatic. After three days, the new family went home. For three weeks, everything went smoothly. The baby was a good eater and a good sleeper. But there was a problem.

Maria couldn't understand why she was crying so easily. And she was so bone-tired. She just didn't know that having a baby would be so much work.

One evening Bryan arrived home from work to find Maria crying in the living room and the baby crying in the bedroom. He took care of the baby first, then he sat down and put his arms around Maria.

"What's going on here?" It looks like a cyclone hit this place. Are you all right?"

"Oh Bryan, I wish we had never had the baby. I just can't go on like this."

A week later, at Maria's one month check-up, she and Bryan related what was happening to Maria. Dr. Maxwell wasn't the least bit surprised. "You have a classic case of post-partum depression, Maria. There are several ways to approach this problem...."

Most of these people recover from these occasional bouts of depression, although the same woman may have depression years later when fired from a job, when she is going through a divorce, or when diagnosed as having a chronic illness.

IDENTIFYING SEVERE DEPRESSION

There are several signs which suggest a major or severe depression. These are:

1. Feelings of sadness lasting too long in relation to the precipitating event.
2. Changes in sleep patterns, such as sleeping too much or very little.
3. Listlessness; little or no energy.
4. Lowered level of alertness and a decreased ability to concentrate.
5. Feelings of guilt.
6. Thoughts of or attempts to commit suicide.
7. Problems with eating, either too much or too little.
8. A sense of worthlessness.
9. Sexual problems.

USING MEDICINE FOR DEPRESSION

In addition to seeing a professional counselor, your physician may prescribe anti-depressant medications to help you. Anti-depressants have many side-effects, such as drowsiness or the feeling of having a hangover. Report any of these to your doctor so that he can alter the dose or change the medicine. Do not take it upon yourself to take more, less, or to discontinue the medication.

WHEN TO INTERVENE

At its worst, depression can lead to thoughts of suicide. Take the word of a potential suicide victim as gospel. *Do not try to humor him or talk him out of his depression or problem.* Threats to commit suicide are very serious, and *you should intervene.* Use your local suicide hot-line. If you are thinking about ending your own life, or know someone else who is, call for help right away.

There are other reasonable times to intervene as well. One, of course, would be if the person were committing bodily harm to himself or to another person. It is frightening to place a friendship on the line by calling for help, but take the time to consider the consequences if you don't.

ONE LAST WORD

Depression can generally be treated. If you or someone you care about is suffering from depression, step forward and get assistance.

It is difficult, if not impossible, to treat one's own depression. Do not let feelings of shame or fear keep you from getting the treatment you need and deserve. Even though you may never have had a problem like this before, the likelihood of having a bout with depression increases significantly once you are diagnosed as being chronically ill. Depression is a serious, hidden hazard of chronic conditions that merits prompt, professional attention.

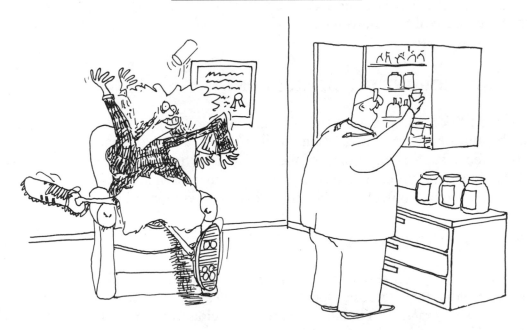

Just nod, Mrs. Livingstone, if you think that anti-depressant is too strong.

BLESSED ARE THE CAREGIVERS

WHO IS A CAREGIVER?

Some of the illnesses discussed in this book may render the sufferer less able to care for himself. For some, "being cared for" is the most humiliating part of an illness. There's no way—and no reason—to sugar-coat this type of dependent relationship, so I want to help you understand it.

A caregiver is any person who takes primary care of another person, either permanently or temporarily. Usually, it is a relationship for which there has been no planning.

Anyone can become a caregiver. Most people have had some experience giving care, at least short-term.

Terry broke her ankle on Tuesday playing basketball in the gym. It was a simple fracture, and, after casting her ankle, Dr. Dixon admonished, "No walking or weight-bearing until Friday."

Back at home, Terry's mother settled her on the couch. Soon the demands began.

"Mom, can you please change the channel?"
"Mom, I'm really hungry. Can I have some lunch?"
"Mom, I spilled my drink all over the couch!"
"Hey, Mom! Can you please get my books for me?"

And so on and so on. . . .

Terry's mother (and the rest of her family) was placed in the role of giving care to Terry on short notice. But they didn't mind. Forty-eight hours isn't very long.

There are other instances when caregiving is very short-lived. It may be more dramatic, but it usually ends quickly. Consider Liam's problem:

A severe case of stomach flu hit Katherine one night after she arrived home after minor surgery. For the first few hours, she was able to rush to the bathroom. But soon, in her weakened state, she vomited and had diarrhea in her bed. She was mortified. Her husband Liam reassured her as best he could.

Katherine was barely able to lift her head. All night long she soiled her bed and vomited. Liam knew that in several hours the flu would be over. Gently he soothed her and cared for her. The washer ran all night and the stench in the room was nearly unbearable. It was a long night, but by morning the worst of the flu had passed.

These situations are short-lived, and therefore easier to manage. The longer the *duration* of the dependency, the more difficult the caregiving relationship will be.

> **"**We make a living by what we get, but we make a life by what we give. **"**
>
> ——ROYLE FORUM

WHY IS A CAREGIVER NEEDED?

When a person cannot live independently, help is needed.

Because of the nature of their chronic condition, some people may find that their overall physical condition is deteriorating. It is with great sadness that a loss of ability is acknowledged. After all, who is willing to admit that he can no longer drive? Walk? Go to the store? Prepare his own meals? Toilet himself and take care of other personal needs?

Accepting care isn't easy, even if the person who needs the care realizes he can no longer function as before. Letting someone take over your care can feel dehumanizing and humiliating.

THE NEED IS INFREQUENT AT FIRST

Often, in the beginning, only occasional help is needed.

Shirley could cook her own meals, but she couldn't take a bath or shampoo her hair alone. Her daughter came in three times a week to help her with personal care chores.

Before too long, however, Shirley couldn't work or stand in the kitchen long enough to cook regularly, either. Her daughter noticed that her mother was preparing only the most simple meals, and finally was eating only toast and cold canned food. The whole family worried that she lived alone.

THE NEED SHIFTS TO FULL CARE

Shirley can no longer care for herself. The reasons don't matter. Now someone else has to assume her care. The need has shifted from partial assistance to almost full care. Somehow, someone will have to assume the full-time care of this person. Who will make the decision to intervene and help Shirley? Who will assume her care?

HOW DOES A PERSON BECOME A CAREGIVER?

There are really only two ways by which a person becomes a caregiver: By decision or by default.

A caregiver may *decide* to help. *Wanting* to help and *being able* to help may be different answers to the same question: Can *you* help take care of this person? Again, the longer the care will be required, the harder this decision is.

A caregiver can decide that yes, there will be enough time, energy, money, and patience to help. It usually isn't a question of enough love, although outsiders often see it that way. Many people in this position are confused by guilt and feelings of obligation that are hard to sort out. In the end, it doesn't matter what the neighbors think or the rest of the family expects, but rather what is workable for the recipient of the care and the caregiver.

A caregiving relationship that is thought through in advance has a good chance of success because everyone involved knows what to expect and most of the difficulties have been anticipated. This is true regardless of the caregiver's position as a family member, friend, paraprofessional, or professional, and whether the caregiver is paid or unpaid.

> Georgianna's Aunt Molly fell and fractured her hip. After some time in the hospital her doctor was ready to release her. But unless she had help, he would not let her go home.

> Georgianna adored Aunt Molly and immediately offered her home during her aunt's convalescence. She knew that as soon as her aunt was healed, she would move back into her apartment and resume her fiercely independent lifestyle.

Georgianna made a conscious decision to help her aunt for all the right reasons. So did Rachel with her husband, Joshua:

> Rachel's beloved husband, Joshua, developed Lou Gehrig's disease. The illness affected him very quickly. It seemed that one day he was a practicing dentist, and the next he was wheelchair bound.

> Rachel immediately assumed the care of her husband. After all, she loved him, and she thought it couldn't be all that difficult. She may not have known what she was getting into, but Rachel chose to care for Joshua. Even if someone told her how difficult giving care would be, she would have done it anyway.

As close friends, Hilda and Emily were also able to arrange a mutually satisfying caregiving relationship.

> Hilda and Emily were life-long friends and next-door neighbors. Hilda developed Alzheimer's Disease. As the months wore on, her symptoms became more severe. Emily spent most of each day with her friend.

> As it became more and more apparent that Hilda needed full-time care, her family became desperate. Funds were limited and the family lived 2,000 miles away.

Everyone was relieved when Emily offered to be responsible for Hilda's care. She would sell her home and move in with her friend. In exchange she had no living expenses and was paid a small salary.

CAREGIVING BY DEFAULT

Most of the horror stories about caregiving—including abusive, guilt-laden, and financially disasterous relationships—are rooted in caregiving situations where one or more of the people involved were unwilling participants. These are the caregiving situations that developed or "just happened" because "there just wasn't anyone else" or "there just wasn't any other way."

A caregiver can find himself or herself in this situation because of limited financial resources, geographic limitations, a family commitment, lack of anyone else to do the job, or a hundred other reasons. This also occurs when short-term caregiving unexpectedly becomes long-term. Like it or not, these caregivers have to make the best of a bad situation. Back to Georgianna and her Aunt Molly:

> Aunt Molly was recovering beautifully from her hip injury. Unfortunately, two weeks before she was due to move back into her apartment, she had a severe stroke.

> It never occurred to Georgianna as the ambulance pulled away that she would literally become her aunt's lifeline. Once Aunt Molly was well enough to go home, she and Georgianna would have to face facts: Her aunt could not live alone again—ever.

> Georgianna felt honor-bound to take her aunt into her home. After all, she was the only close relative. And so she became Aunt Molly's long-term caregiver.

The good news is that some of these relationships become highly successful. Surprisingly for everyone involved, many people end up caring about each other very deeply as people, not as problems or adversaries.

The person who accepts caregiving by default usually has no other choice. It seems, at the time, to be the only solution to a very difficult problem. Regardless of the genuine feelings of affection for the person needing care, the caregiver is placed in a difficult position. Against his or her will, the caregiver may have to share the illness to the extent of personal sacrifice or hardship. This pressure gets the relationship off to a poor start, and can keep generating negative feelings.

A default relationship would not be as troublesome if our Western culture venerated the extended family more. In cultures that revere both distant cousins and great-grandparents, taking in one or more family member is not as big a concern. Because there are more people in the house, caregiving does not fall on just one or two people, either.

In any case, because we are chronically ill, we are the least welcome in *any* culture. We are the most trouble to take care of. We don't get better. We usually don't die quickly enough to justify our caregiver's heroic endurance. We don't contribute evenly or equally. We just force our problems on those around us. Those of us who have had to depend upon other people for caregiving know how difficult it is to build and maintain good relationships with them.

Our guilt, plus our caregiver's guilt and resentment, particularly in a default situation, can lead to a complex, stressful relationship. We can help this situation if we can learn to empathize with the caregiver.

UNDERSTANDING THE CAREGIVER

By now, you should realize that the romantic notions of caregiving conceal a more grim reality. Caregiving is *not* always selfless love transferred to another individual in need. In fact, caregiving can be difficult and exhausting.

There is little glory involved in being a caregiver. It requires a great deal of guts. No type of care is exempt from the caregiver's able hands. No chore is too basic. When total care is required, the responsibilities may range in a single day from doing the wash or cleaning up a bowl of spilled soup to giving a shower or removing a bowel impaction.

Caregivers quickly learn to eat when the person they are caring for eats, to sleep when he sleeps, and to do the chores in a mad rush between it all.

Few caregivers are praised. Few want glory. Most want just a little more help and a good night's sleep.

Certainly many people who care for a loved one would not think of having it any other way. They care so much, and it hurts to see their loved one suffer.

Still, there is a considerable toll taken from these people. It doesn't matter how much you love the person you are caring for, a caregiver is still likely to become exhausted and drained. It is not an easy job.

SOMETIMES, CAREGIVERS FEEL TRAPPED AND ANGRY

It is difficult for a caregiver to separate himself physically from the care receiver. Often, there is little or no opportunity to do so. Some caregivers feel guilty to admit it, but after a while, they feel trapped by their new responsibilities.

In the beginning, it may not seem difficult to be "on call" 24 hours a day, seven days a week. But soon, each day seems a week long. As exhaustion creeps in and the caregiver feels more and more alone, he may begin to feel tremendous anger. This may result in an outpouring of fury and resentment.

Anger is a normal emotion, and it is certainly understandable in this situation. However, if left to fester, it will become uncontrollable and begin to affect every other aspect of the caregiving relationship. The internal stress the caregiver feels may cause him to become ill himself.

Surprisingly, the problem of anger becomes even more difficult to deal with if the person receiving the care is still mentally capable. When this is the case, overwhelming guilt on the part of both caregiver and care recipient can ensue. After all, the recipient never intended to be the object of someone else's care. Guilt seems to beget guilt.

"How," Eunice reasons, "do I dare feel mad when it's Charlie who is suffering. He's always so apologetic. . . ."

STAY PATIENT AND GET COMFORTABLE

To the caregivers and care receivers reading this, I implore you to be patient with each other. It's no easy task to assume the full care of another person. Regardless of how idealistic you are, you will find there are no easy answers.

You both need to begin by expecting the best and preparing for the worst. Give courage to each other. There will be good times, too. When all the chores are done and you are both well-rested, remember to do something nice for each other. Keep working to make your relationship better.

> **“**One of the signs of maturity is a healthy respect for reality—a respect that manifests itself in the level of one's aspirations and in the accuracy of one's assessment of the difficulties which separate the facts of today from the bright hopes of tomorrow. **”**
>
> ___ROBERT H. DAVIES

Whether by decision or default, you are both stuck with each other for now. Perhaps the suggestions on the following pages will help each of you make the best of the situation, starting with a few things you need to think about when beginning the caregiving arrangement.

Give each other time to come to terms with the other and come to grips with the dynamics of the new relationship. The caregiver needs to find out what to do and how to do it. The recipient needs to learn to allow the care. These are not easy lessons—for either of you!

You may be surprised that the guidelines for each of you are similar. Share them with your counterpart, and use them to start your own discussions.

SUGGESTIONS FOR THE CAREGIVER

Include the other person as much as possible in your daily plans, no matter how small the involvement may seem. This could include discussing a breakfast selection, deciding what to watch on TV, or talking about whether to wear a blue or brown shirt. These may seem trivial to you, but when a person's world has narrowed to the confines of a few rooms, being included is extremely important to his self-esteem.

Don't assume anything, especially when it involves the needs or emotions of another person.

Develop a personal support system so that any anger or frustration you feel is not vented on the person for whom you are caring.

Ask the person what he wants. He or she is not an object nor a "problem." Let him continue to have input into his own life.

Treat the care recipient with dignity and respect. You are dealing with another human being. That person never wanted to be in this dependent relationship, either.

Learn to prioritize. Sometimes a waxed kitchen floor just isn't as important as enjoying a beautiful day together.

Communicate, communicate, communicate. If ever it was important to be honest and open, it's now. I recognize that not all communication will be interesting during your day, so learn to deal well with what communication there is.

❝ Hope is the dream of a man awake. ❞

——Matthew Prior

SUGGESTIONS FOR THE CARE RECIPIENT

Be grateful. Don't lose sight of the fact that another person is working hard to care for your needs, both physical and emotional. Say thank you, and don't be stingy with positive feedback.

Don't assume anything. If your caregiver is crabby one day, don't automatically assume it is because of you. At least ask. Your caregiver has feelings, too, and a life beyond you. Reach out—maybe you can help.

Communicate your needs, but do so without "giving orders." This person is providing a service, but he or she is not your servant. When you find that you have unmet needs, be sure to express yourself as an adult. If ever it was important to talk, openly and honestly, it's now. Communicate, communicate, communicate.

Get cleaned up and dressed each and every day. Stay proud of yourself by looking as good as you can. You may not look as good as you used to, but you can still maintain your pride.

Stop complaining. When friends come by, don't bore them with the details of how miserable you are. If you want them to stay friends, be as pleasant as you are able.

Treat your caregiver with dignity and respect. Remember that you, too, are dealing with another human being. Your caregiver may have unmet needs, too. Mutual respect provides the bridges you both need to get over the rough spots ahead.

"I believe that every person must act according to the dictates of his conscience. I feel that the capacity to care is the thing that gives life its deepest significance and meaning. "

——PABLO CASALS

MAKING DECISIONS AND CHANGES

Periodically, every caregiver needs to step back and assess his or her role in the relationship. These are the questions that have to be asked:

1. Are you happy? Are you at least satisfied?
2. Are you doing all the caregiving? Why?
3. Can you get some help?
4. Do you have any options available if you become ill or need to be hospitalized?
5. Can the care recipient be left alone for any period of time?
6. Do you completely understand the recipient's current medical condition and what his needs are?
7. Are you repelled by his medical or physical condition?
8. Who is meeting your physical needs?
9. Who is meeting your emotional needs? Is there a support group for others in similar situations?
10. Are you angry? Do you feel resentful?
11. Are you taking out your anger on the person for whom you are caring?
12. Do you have a friend, physician, or clergyman with whom you can be brutally honest?

13. Are you allowing yourself to have a separate life away from your charge, or has your task become your whole life?
14. Do you have a job or activities away from home?
15. By now you realize that you are "working" a 24-hour day. If something were to happen to change the circumstances, such as a worsening of the physical condition or even the death of the person receiving the care, would you be able to put your life back together?

NO PERFECT SOLUTIONS

Every caregiver needs a break, but relief is often limited. Here are some suggestions which may help:

1. Can a friend or relative relieve you a few hours one or two days each week? In this way, you can have a well-earned break from the daily rigors of caregiving.
2. Do you have the financial resources to hire a caregiver for a few hours each day? Teenagers and senior citizens are good at this job, and the added income is welcome. If you can't pay, perhaps you can barter for services, e.g., "I'll bake you three loaves of bread for every two hours you fill in for me."
3. Can you arrange for extra help from any social service agency in your community? What about a visiting nurse?
4. Ask the disease-oriented associations, such as the multiple sclerosis society, if they can suggest places to call for help. While you're at it, request information about the loan or rental of wheelchairs, walkers, and so forth.
5. What about getting a job? (Don't laugh!) Can you work full or part-time, and hire someone else to take over your at-home job, at least for a few hours each day? You may pay most of your salary to the person you have hired, but you are more likely to be happy if you have a change of pace and are not required to give of yourself all day.
6. Have you considered trading afternoons with someone else who is providing care, too? The care required may be similar, but the emotional cost is different.
7. Have you found a coping or support group for caregivers? These are available, and it will help immensely to talk about your common

problems. If one is not available, how about starting one yourself?

8. What about assigning some time, once a week, to other relatives, so that you can run errands and take care of your other personal needs?

9. Try to keep yourself interesting and developing as a person. Develop new hobbies and interests, if possible. Keep up on current events. You will be more proud of yourself and you won't stagnate intellectually.

10. What about investigating a day-care situation for disabled people? Some nursing homes, rehabilitation centers, and neighborhood houses provide this valuable service.

11. If you need to get away for awhile or become ill yourself, some nursing homes provide short-term care.

NURSING HOMES

Finally, a few words about permanently changing the place of residence for the person who requires the care. Yes, I mean a nursing home. This may become necessary, for example, when:

1. The medical condition of the care recipient changes so that one person cannot adequately deliver all the care required.

2. The mental or physical health of the caregiver changes.

3. Caregiving in the home is no longer a viable option for one reason or another.

A nursing home should by no means be considered a last resort. Most are run by caring, qualified people who deal daily with the same types of problems you are coping with. As a matter of fact, what may seem like a crisis to you may be commonplace to them. If you genuinely want the best quality of care, nursing homes must be considered.

You have many options when it comes to admission to a nursing home. You can probably visit every day, and stay as long as you like. You may be able to take your friend or relative home overnight, or out for a drive or dinner.

It's not easy to place someone you love into a nursing home, but sometimes it really is the most viable choice.

ALLOW TIME FOR YOURSELF

I've said it before and I'll say it again, "If you don't take care of yourself, there will be nothing left for anyone else."

Giving and receiving long-term care by choice or default is always difficult. When you find yourself in either role, allow time for yourself. Work to make your relationship with your "partner in care" more supportive and constructive. Keep your sense of perspective and your sense of humor, and you can make the most of the situation. Good luck!

RESTING, RELAXING, AND RELATED CONCERNS

What a blow to your ego! When you were younger, or well, or both, you ran, took stairs two at a time, and otherwise took your good health for granted. It requires a tremendous adjustment to realize that you need a lot more rest and sleep now. If you do not allow yourself more rest, your body simply cannot perform at even minimal levels. Most of us are finding it absolutely essential to schedule a nap or rest period every day.

READING YOUR BODY'S SIGNALS

Even the simple chores of daily living can be insurmountable if you are chronically ill. Rolling out of bed, washing up, getting dressed, negotiating the stairs, or preparing a meal can be exhausting. You are probably discovering the importance of reading the new signals your body sends you when you are getting too tired. Learn to recognize fatigue before it catches up with you. If you reach the point of serious exhaustion or, as I call it, the point of no return, you risk serious physical harm. If you know you have pushed yourself too far and cannot do another thing, swallow your pride and take the rest you know you need—before you cause an accident for yourself or someone else.

PREPARE TO REST

Resting means more than making a cup of coffee and sitting down at the kitchen table with the morning newspaper. It also means more than leaning against the wall in the restroom at work! A real rest restores all of your muscles and your psychological stamina; sitting or standing still requires both. It is better to get quality rest in a shorter period of time, rather than struggle along by grabbing a few minutes here and there.

Make a habit of resting at a particular time and in a particular place every day. Those at home will find this advice easier to follow than those who work. You may have to improvise a technique on the job or wait and rest when you arrive home. But do include a resting period in your daily routine. If you cannot function well physically, you won't have any "extra" energy left to share with your family or friends.

RESTING ISN'T EASY

Resting that really helps you requires more attention than you might think. You must remove all physical and mental stress and pressure. This is easier said than done. Even though your body desperately needs and wants to rest, your thoughts will often continue racing ahead unless you train yourself to "let go."

Before you lie down, prepare a comfortable resting area and darken the room. Make sure that there is support underneath all parts of your body. If you have pain in one or more areas, place pillows underneath to provide extra support. The best position for rest is on your back. If some of you find this position too painful, check with your doctor about placing a pillow beneath your knees to offer more support. (Some medical conditions prohibit resting with bent knees.)

To begin, keep your eyes open and clear your mind by choosing a specific spot to stare at. It could be a picture on a wall, a light fixture, a crack in the ceiling, or anything else that you can focus on. Continue to focus on your target until it begins to change shape. Do you remember ever lying on your back in sweet-smelling grass looking for shapes in the clouds? Conjure up the sheer pleasure of the moment. Remember the smells, the sounds, and the feeling of complete contentment? Use that kind of memory to help relax.

Next, allow your eyes to close. Be sure your body is very still. Take four *very* slow breaths. You will find that you are already calming down and your body is beginning to sink into the cushions underneath you.

As you continue to take slow, deep breaths, concentrate on allowing each part of your body to relax, one by one. Begin with your toes. Wiggle them, letting the tension go. Flex your knees a little. Let your lower back drop flat, letting all that stress and pressure float away. Relax your shoulders and arms, all the way down to your fingers. Now relax those tense neck and head muscles.

If you do this successfully, you will find yourself in the twilight zone that just precedes sleep, or drifting from relaxing rest into sleep.

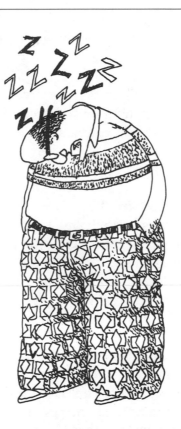

Not a good way to rest!

While you rest, focus your imagination on sounds and sights which are pleasing to you, like a beautiful waterfall or birds singing. Perhaps thinking of yourself in a boat, floating on a river, or swinging in a hammock works for you. Don't hesitate to indulge yourself. Some people prefer to listen to soft, restful music.

Stay in this relaxed position as long as you feel it is doing you some good. I try to set a limit before I lie down so I don't fall asleep and upset my sleep schedule. After I set my internal "alarm clock," I can rest completely, without worry or guilt, because I have prepared myself to wake up refreshed. If you don't have a good sense of time when you rest, have someone check on you after a period of time, or set a clock radio to go on at a low volume at a certain time.

Many people need to repeat this process more than once a day. There are no hard and fast rules. Learn to be sensitive to your own needs. Soon, you'll wonder how you ever managed before.

Another method of relaxation is worth trying if you tend to be tense. First tighten a set of muscles, hold them taut for five seconds, then release. For example, tighten your forehead, hold for five seconds, then relax. Do the same with your arms, then your shoulders, and so on throughout your body.

YOU NEED TO RELAX, TOO

In addition to planning periods of rest, you need to learn how to find time to *relax* during the day. Resting and relaxing are different. Whether or not you are chronically ill, you need to get away from the tedium of a day-to-day routine. Relaxation provides this essential break. Of course, chronic illness puts some limits on what form your relaxation takes. As you regroup your thoughts about what you can and cannot do, you'll discover a wide range of activities which can be quite enjoyable. These diversions or distractions may be less strenuous, but they can still be interesting and challenging enough to stimulate you. Think about playing a musical instrument, collecting stamps, doing handicrafts, or reading.

Your illness might reveal talents you have neglected or never recognized before. If skiing had been a special interest before your illness, you may discover that photographing skiers as they come down the slopes can provide a satisfying and creative outlet for this interest. The point is to look for alternative ways of relaxing and enjoying yourself.

" A man without a plan for the day is lost before he starts. "

——LEWIS E. BENDELE

TRY KEEPING A JOURNAL

Another way to relax is to keep a daily journal in which you write down your private thoughts, successes, failures, and plans. It doesn't require as much exertion as racquetball, and even if you can't write or type anymore, you can always use a tape recorder.

Keeping a journal can contribute to your mental relaxation in three ways. First, it serves as a sounding board. It's often a relief to unburden your innermost thoughts without shifting them to someone else's shoulders. Second, it provides a satisfying way to mark time; you can graphically see your small successes accumulating. Most important, if you get into the habit of writing in a journal, or even writing a list, you can lay to rest those thoughts which keep you from getting needed rest or sleep. If you feel uncomfortable keeping a journal, write down your thoughts and throw the paper away in a few days.

HOW DO YOU SPELL RELAX?

Dr. Howard Shapiro, a nationally known psychiatrist who has a chronic illness himself, has one of the best definitions of genuine relaxation I've come across. He bases his comprehensive understanding of relaxation on the letters of the word "relaxes." Each letter stands for some aspect of the total relaxation we need. He has graciously given me permission to share his definition.

R: Rest, relax, and recreate regularly. This does not mean just on weekends or holidays, but all the time, as a new life pattern. Now is the time to drop your workaholic tendencies. If you have neglected to incorporate "R" into your life so far, it is essential now that chronic illness has entered the picture.

E: Exercise! Not all of you can get out and jog or play tennis, but you should do what you can, at least several times a week, even if you are bound to a bed or wheelchair. Ask your doctor to help you develop an exercise plan suited to your illness. Activity is important, even if it is just range of motion exercises.

L: Laughter can be crucial for your survival. You may be familiar with Norman Cousins, former editor of *Saturday Review,* who used laughter as the key part of his successful attempt to reach a remission of his illness. The same treatment can help us deal with our chronic illness. Laughter doesn't just make you feel good; it also causes you to take deep, relaxing breaths and, for a short time, it clears your mind of other thoughts and emotions. And laughter begets laughter. What a wonderful habit to develop!

A: Affection, both given and received. Share yourself! Pet a puppy, hug a child, love your spouse. Equally important, learn to ask for and receive affection in whatever way you feel comfortable. Don't be shy—make it a constant in your life.

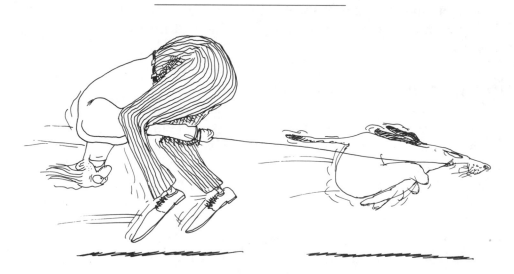

Remedy for lethargy.

X: Exchange negative thoughts for positive thoughts. Dwell on what you can change, not on what you can't. Think about how well you can be instead of how ill you might be.

E: Educate yourself about your chronic illness. And don't educate only yourself. Take it upon yourself to gently and slowly educate those around you who care about your well-being.

S: Socialize with and offer support to others as much as your condition allows, plus a little more. If you keep yourself busy, you'll have less time to dwell on your pain and illness. It's hard to concentrate on two things at once. A particularly good way of keeping busy is to use your experiences to provide encouragement and support to others with a similar condition. By helping others, you help yourself even more.

Keep Dr. Shapiro's list in mind and get your daily share of r-e-l-a-x-e-s!

❝ Sleep is nature's way of readying your body for a new tomorrow. ❞

—Sefra Pitzele

SLEEPING AND INSOMNIA

In addition to rest and relaxation, you need to get sufficient sleep. You probably need more because of your illness, yet find it harder to get because of your discomfort and new routines. This problem is not confined to the chronically ill. One-third of all adults complain to their doctors about insomnia. It's a serious physical ailment that can wear you down and make you susceptible to illness and accidents.

There are three types of insomnia. *Initial* insomnia occurs when a person goes to bed and cannot fall asleep. *Intermittent* insomnia comes and goes during the night, and appears to affect the elderly more often, especially if there is a concurrent physical problem. *Terminal* insomnia describes the sleep problems of a person who falls asleep quickly and awakens after only a few hours of sleep. He cannot get back to sleep for the rest of the night.

When a person is deprived of sleep for a long time, his perceptions alter, and he may even hallucinate. Reaction time becomes more erratic, making it dangerous to drive or perform a physical activity. Efficiency, judgment, attentiveness, and the ability to complete tasks are diminished. The person who is not getting enough sleep may even suffer a basic change in personality, becoming more negative, disinterested, and perhaps seriously depressed. Sleep-deprived people may be misdiagnosed because of the mental and physical changes caused by lack of sleep.

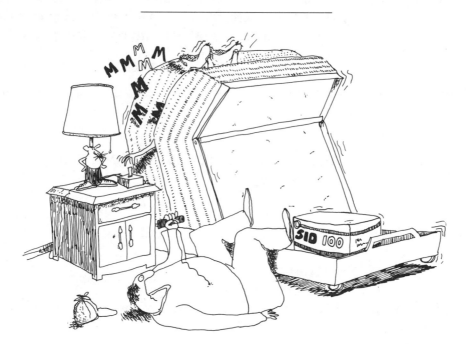

Herman's fourth attempt to fix the electric bed fails.

COPING WITH SLEEPLESSNESS AT NIGHTTIME

Most of you who suffer from chronic illness understand what I call "aloneness in the night." Hours seem longer during the night and your pain seems to double. Your house or apartment is very quiet. If you are married, you are reluctant to bother your spouse. Often, no one else in the family knows that you are awake; you wander around the house trying not to make noise, knowing that it will be difficult to get through the next day with little or no sleep. A vicious cycle can trap you. First, you can't sleep. Then you lie awake worrying that you can't sleep. And then you're exhausted the next day.

Try surrendering yourself to the comfortable and familiar; don't forget Grandmother's tried and true methods for falling asleep, like a long warm bath, reading a relaxing book, or drinking a glass of warm milk.

Massage can also help you feel relaxed and sleepy. If no one is available to massage your back and neck, you can do it yourself, as long as your joints are able to exert or stand the pressure.

Once you are settled in bed, try to use the skills you have learned to help you rest. Visualize a relaxing image. Listen to soft music. Invent sleep games such as counting backward from 200. I tell myself that if I lose my place, I have to begin again. You may have to perform these feats several times before falling asleep, but it gets easier.

Be careful of what you eat and drink before bedtime. Most people who have sleep problems quickly learn to avoid products that contain caffeine, such as coffee, hot chocolate, or cola products. What most people don't know, however, is that caffeine can act as a stimulant for up to four hours—so drinking coffee at six may make it difficult to get to sleep at 10 o'clock. Make sure to read the ingredients label on soft drinks and other products you eat before bedtime.

If these techniques don't work, take another look at your daily resting habits. Are you getting enough rest? It is possible to be *too* tired to sleep well.

KEEP A LIST

Sometimes, persistent worry and anxiety defeat even our best efforts to get to sleep. In the book, *A Natural Sleep*, Dr. David Viscott is quoted as saying, "To acquire the right attitude for dealing with insomnia, you must understand that you can't cope with all your problems at the same time."

In other words, try not to make a habit of taking worries to bed with you. Sleep comes easier when personal conflicts are resolved. Don't go to bed angry at yourself or anyone else. Problems are rarely solved alone in the dark of the night.

Although your problems may seem overwhelming in the wee hours, I have learned a simple way to cut them down to size. Before getting into bed, write down all your problems, beginning with the biggest and ending with the smallest. Think about possible solutions and list those, too. Writing down your plan of action ensures that you won't forget about it tomorrow. It also gives you a sense that you have taken a definite step forward toward solving your problems; you don't have to think about your worries anymore tonight.

It may also help you relax and sleep if you list your schedule for the next day. Many people with chronic illness, especially those with significant pain, find mornings difficult to face. By listing those chores or activities which must be done, you are giving yourself the mental boost necessary to get out of bed.

If you sometimes find yourself with empty mornings, create an "emergency activity" list. Put it aside and use it only when you are desperate for something to do. This list could include chores you try to forget, such as straightening out cupboards, cleaning the basement, or reorganizing your workbench. Most of you will be able to come up with something to do to avoid the "emergency" list!

SOLVE YOUR SLEEP PROBLEM CREATIVELY

Although my own sleep problem is not completely solved, let me share my techniques with you. First, after I have determined that I am not going to fall asleep normally, I leave my bed and move to the sofa. If I am really not sleepy, I will read or listen to the radio for a while. Then I purposefully turn out the lights and tell myself that while I do not have to sleep, I *do* have to clear my mind and at least rest. Then, I generally use one or more of the relaxation techniques I described earlier. Often I fall asleep just because I play that old child's game of telling myself that I do not have to go to sleep!

Whether or not you use any of these techniques is strictly a matter of what works for you. It does not matter how you rest and sleep, but it is important that you do it regularly. You cannot cope with your illness or your life in general unless you have gotten the rest, relaxation, and sleep that you need and deserve!

IF YOU NEED MORE HELP, ASK

If you reach a point where you cannot deal with insomnia through your own efforts, check with your doctor. A hidden problem may be the cause, or perhaps a medicine is producing a side effect that is keeping you awake at night.

If your physician does not find a specific medical reason for your insomnia, he may prescribe a short program incorporating a sleeping medicine to break the "no-sleep" cycle. In addition, he may suggest relaxation therapy, which is a more formal method of learning to relax, and may include biofeedback or hypnotism. To implement any of these suggestions, you will need the help of a professional. Your doctor can recommend the necessary specialist.

RELAXATION THERAPY, HYPNOSIS, AND BIOFEEDBACK

I have learned all three methods, and by and large, they stand me in good stead. I use the skills I learned in relaxation therapy several times a day. If I am having a hard time sleeping, I keep working with it until I am asleep.

There is a very fine line between relaxation therapy and hypnosis. I first became interested in hypnosis as a way to deal with pain. My first efforts to try it were terrifying. I was so afraid of losing control and making an absolute fool of myself that I had fits of nervous giggling during the first few sessions. The psychologist must have thought me quite strange! Once I got used to the terminology and the wonderful feelings of complete relaxation, I began to realize that there was nothing to fear.

There are many reasons to learn hypnosis, but pain and anxiety control certainly top the list. Ask your doctor if hypnosis would help. Learning self-hypnosis is another way to re-gain control of yourself.

Let me dispel some of the common fears and misconceptions about hypnosis for those of you who may want to try it. Rest assured that you will not act like a character in a Las Vegas stageshow! You will not do anything that is completely out of character. You will, however, be able to clear your mind of all extraneous thoughts and zero-in on total relaxation. If you want to move from rest to the stage of sleep, hypnosis or deep relaxation can make it possible.

I worked for a while on biofeedback to see if I could learn to raise the temperature in my very cold fingers. Biofeedback is a method of mentally controlling one's own bodily functions with visual or audible feedback. The book, *A Natural Sleep,* includes Dr. Peter Hauri's version of the five basic steps of biofeedback. Here is a simplified version of the process:

1. Decide what to measure. For example, you may wish to measure your ability to relax your jaw muscles.
2. Learn how the biofeedback (measurement) device works.
3. Learn by trial and error what you must do to change the feedback. Your method may be a certain way of channeling or focusing your mental or emotional energy. Your feedback to yourself may be visible or audible.
4. Practice. Success begets success, and it gets easier and easier to show positive results.
5. Finally, you learn what to do within yourself to create the change at will, and the biofeedback machine can be removed.

It is important to recognize that biofeedback does not hurt, and that even though the biofeedback machine uses electricity, you will not get shocked. Biofeedback is an easy way to learn to change how you deal with pain or negative behavior patterns. The good habits you learn on a biofeedback machine can then be put to use for the rest of your life.

INCORPORATE RELAXATION INTO YOUR LIFE

My mother always used to say, "All work and no play makes Jack a dull boy." To twist it a bit, "All seriousness and no fun makes an ill person boring!" You and your illness are not two separate entities. You must learn to live with and merge your illness into your everyday life. Think of circles overlapping in many areas. You are still in the center, as the same person, but there are areas here and there which are touched by your chronic illness. In order to survive, it becomes necessary to identify emotionally, intellectually, and physically with your illness without becoming overwhelmed. Just as you have made various other adjustments throughout your life, you and your family must now adjust to your illness, and incorporate it as an important, but *small* part of your lives.

Taking resting, relaxing, and sleeping seriously will ensure that you are mentally and physically prepared to cope and change. You are already fighting one battle with your body—don't let another get started!

You must find your own way to adapt your new self to old situations, for it is the ability to adapt that allows you to live more comfortably with illness.

With your ability to change and your new knowledge of how to rest and relax, you will be able to form new habits and get on with the business of living.

> **"The soul is dyed the color of its leisure thoughts."**
>
> ——DEAN INGE

A WHISPER IN THE NIGHT

Sex and your sexuality

PILLOW TALK

A tiny whisper in the night . . .
Do you want to? Well, turn out the light.

Will illness keep me forever from holding her?
From knowing the smell of her skin and the joy of enfolding her?

A fingertip stroking a cheek—gently caressing a chin.
Illness can bring us closer . . . we have only to begin.

—SEFRA PITZELE, 1984

A chronic, restrictive, medical condition can have a significant impact on your sexual activities. "Obviously," you say, thinking about people you know who are paralyzed from the waist down or whose medications cause them to feel uncomfortable much of the time. But the impact goes beyond the physical effects of a chronic condition. What about the psychological effect of your illness on, for example, your sense of self-esteem? And what about the subsequent changes in your desire and ability to participate in sexual activities?

When you're 30 pounds heavier because of the cortisone you have to take, or when you're sure your spouse deeply resents every single thing about your chronic illness, sexual intimacy is naturally more stressful.

This chapter is about sexuality, and the special situations you may face because of your chronic illness. Don't give up yet—I offer some very specific information and practical approaches to solving some of the predictable problems related to your illness.

This information is for everyone, young or old, well or ill, single or married, who needs more information about sex and sexuality as they relate to a chronic medical condition. Start where you are right now. If sex and sexual feelings were important to you before you became ill, you will want to read this.

WE NEED INTIMACY

We each require different types of intimacy, whether it takes the form of shaking a good friend's hand, slapping a buddy on the back during a ball game, or hugging a child. We all have the need to share the beauty of a sunset, or the pleasure of a long walk with a friend. Many of us have spiritual intimacy in our belief in God. And for many, our most powerful and beautiful feelings of intimacy result from sexual love. Therein lies one of the greatest problems associated with chronic illness.

Chronic illness does not take away a person's desire or appetite for sex. We still need to be caressed and held and fondled. We still need to love and be loved. We still need to have the physical and emotional releases that sex provides. But many of us never anticipated the changes that would alter our tried and true sexual patterns. When these changes occur, we suffer a profound sense of loss.

IS SEX IMPORTANT TO YOU?

There is a problem if you begin to pretend that sex and sexual feelings are no longer important to you when in fact they really are. A relationship, like a fine diamond, is made up of many facets. One part of a relationship, and one part of your own sexuality, is having sexual feelings.

If you let your desire for sex be pushed into the background, another facet of your relationship will be gone. It drifts away, often forever. Before you let that happen, think it through. Is that what you really want?

So what if sex as you knew it before chronic illness is now virtually impossible. You can still compensate, adjust, and improve. Physical affection in a less-demanding form is often as important, if not more important, than sexual intercourse. A smile, a hug, a stroke, a caress, or a pat on the back are often important expressions of sexuality, and may be more affirming. And after all, no one has to make special plans to hug someone.

It has often been said that sex is more cerebral than physical. The pleasure, the warmth, and the intimacy of sex are all recorded and appreciated by the brain. That special feeling two people feel for each other which is demonstrated in the old song, "Little Things Mean a Lot," still matters a great deal. "Touch my hair when you pass my chair. Little things mean a lot." Romance still counts. I urge you to use your imagination.

Regardless of our physical condition, we all need to be sensitive to our own and to other's sexual needs. Since sexuality is intertwined with self-image, and self-image can be intertwined with chronic illness, problems can occur that confuse us and cause us to draw inward.

❝ Learn to like what you are, for you take yourself with you wherever you go. ❞

——SEFRA PITZELE

PHYSICAL CHANGES OCCUR FIRST

We notice physical changes first. Bodies we have been able to count on are now betraying us, inflicting pain and exhaustion at the most unexpected times. Pain can cause fear about sexual performance. Other physical difficulties such as limited range of motion, pain in specific areas in the body, exhaustion, inability to maintain an erection, or lack of lubrication, all add to the problems.

In addition, either you or your partner may now have an altered perception of you. Do you feel fragile? Ugly? Unworthy? Your self-image can change due to pain and loss of ability, or because of deformity caused by the disease or required medications. Some drugs, especially cortisone, can dramatically alter how a person looks.

CHRONIC ILLNESS PRESENTS A NEW PROBLEM—TIMING

The advent of chronic illness makes the timing of sex a new and frequently unanticipated problem. In the past, physical sex was, for most of us, a spontaneous outpouring of affection for our partner. Now, morning stiffness, exhaustion, pain, and all the other limitations of chronic illness place constraints on when and how often we can have sex. These problems may seem overwhelming at first, but common sense, preplanning, and communication can cut them down to size. I particularly want to emphasize the importance of communication. Openness and a willingness to talk honestly are crucial where sexual difficulties are encountered.

Actually, the problem of timing is probably one of the easiest to solve. Clearly there is a greater need to discuss and plan for sex ahead of time. You might also have to consider making love at different times of the day. For example, if you are usually too tired in the evenings, how about in the morning, or before dinner, or whatever time of the day you feel most rested and energetic? Although some of the spontaneity may be gone, that doesn't for a moment mean that the enjoyment is lessened. Anticipation can be a turn-on, too.

Imagine this scenario: Virginia is worried because she and John have not had sex for many weeks. She is no longer able to do all the physical things she used to be capable of and she is in pain much of the time. She is also suffering from the side-effects of drug therapy. Because of these limitations, she is starting to feel that she is unworthy of his affection. In the meantime, her husband desperately wants to have sex with his wife, or at least be cuddled and held. He thinks to himself, "How can I inflict my needs upon her when she is having so many problems of her own? Besides, I'm afraid that I might hurt her and add to her pain. But I miss the intimacy of our sex more than I can say."

Let's listen in on Virginia and John one evening. John's approach is direct and sincere:

"Honey, how about if you and I plan a nice quiet dinner together this Saturday? We can send the kids to your sister's house and have ourselves a little roll in the hay, just like we used to!"

"I guess we really have to sit down and talk about this, John. You may think I've been avoiding sex, and I guess I have. I'm really scared that it will hurt. The pain is so bad in my hips now, I'm afraid I won't be able to enjoy myself. Could we have dinner and then just see how I feel?"

Early on Saturday, Virginia begins to really think about that evening. She very much wants to make love with her husband, but she is scared. "I wonder if I take a pain pill at dinner if it will help me have less discomfort. I'm really going to make an effort to figure this out...it means a lot to me."

Later on that evening: "Dinner was wonderful, John. I haven't felt this relaxed for months. The house is really quiet with the children gone. I think I'm going to take a nice warm bubble bath. Want to join me?"

"In the tub? We haven't done that for years! Move over, lady!"

"I'll wash your back if you'll wash mine."

"I have a better idea. I'll wash your front if you'll wash mine!!!"

To make a long story short, John and Virginia were able to have a warm, close, and rewarding experience. They did make love. Virginia had read in her arthritis booklet, *Living and Loving,* that she could lie on her back and John could support his own body weight. She took a pain pill and relaxed in a hot tub beforehand. Because they opened the doors of communication, they were able to carefully plan for sex. And because they both wanted it, it became very important.

When couples sit down together and talk about this very delicate and often painful topic, they are often surprised to discover how much the other person has missed their former intimacy. One might find that the other needs reassurance of love to help get over feelings of unworthiness. Both soon realize that they need physical affection, but not necessarily physical sex. By sharing their concern, a couple can find a way to enjoy sexual intimacy once again. When the lines of communication have been reestablished in this important area, they may find that their overall life together improves. It will certainly become more complete.

It is important to learn about your body inside and out. Become comfortable with how you look. Stand before a mirror and accept yourself as you are—not as who you wish you could be.

❝ The key is communication—with your partner, your physician, and your best friend. **❞**

——SEFRA PITZELE

RECOGNIZING NORMAL AND ABNORMAL SEXUAL CHANGES IN MEN

Tied up with all the other sensitive feelings about sex is the fear or realization that changes are also occurring as part of our normal aging process.

As men reach their fifth and sixth decade, they may begin to notice changes. Their once strong urinary stream may be less powerful, and they may tend to dribble at the end of urination. Erection might not come as quickly and the penis may not be as hard or firm as in the past.

In addition, the male may be slower to ejaculate, which in some cases is a decided advantage. This is especially true if he has had a history of premature ejaculation. Delay of ejaculation may allow a long time for mutual or self-stimulation.

These are normal physiological changes that occur as men age. Some men complain that it takes them much longer to achieve an erection. Impotence is a term often used in this context to identify both the normal waning of capability for erection and a decreased desire for sex.

Psychological and emotional problems almost always develop when a man becomes impotent (unable to maintain an erection). A tremendous amount of a man's "maleness" is tied up in his ability to "perform" sexually. While a woman doesn't lose the physical capability to make love, it is quite obvious when a man loses that capability—there is no way to fake an erection! When the ability to have intercourse is lost, most men have trouble even talking about it, let alone seeing a doctor.

Impotence is usually caused by one of the following:

1. Medication.
2. Neurological disorder (i.e., multiple sclerosis).
3. Poor circulation.

4. Diabetes.
5. Psychological problems (i.e., anxiety or stress).
6. Physiological problems.

WHOSE CUP IS IT, ANYHOW?

Is it human nature that if there are fifty-nine good minutes in an hour and one bad one, we only remember the bad?

Is my cup half empty or half full?

So why am I sitting here with tears running down my cheeks?

Because it's awfully hard to hang on to the fifty-nine minutes when someone else keeps trying to empty your cup.

I can't and won't allow it. It's my cup.
And I'm going to keep it full of my love for life and with as much happiness as I am capable of producing.

——*Sefra Pitzele, 1984*

It's important not to give up on sex just because impotence has occurred. Talk to your partner, and see a doctor if necessary. Sometimes it's just a matter of identifying an underlying cause, physical or psychological, and eliminating it. If the physical problem does not lend itself to an easy solution, or if you can't change from a medication that causes impotence, then you may wish to see a urologist. He may provide new insights about the extent of the trouble, or suggest surgically implanting a penile prosthesis. The prosthesis is implanted beneath the skin of the penis, and enables the man to penetrate during intercourse.

If after seeing your doctor you still have no way of maintaining an erection, it is critical to understand that sexual activity still does not have to end.

Unfortunately, communication breaks down more often at this time than at any other, and the topic of sex may be permanently buried under silence, avoidance, and anger. Remember that there are many ways to satisfy your partner without penetration, and you can still enjoy the intimacy of fondling, holding, and kissing. You need to talk to each other, openly and honestly, to discover which methods are best for you and your partner.

Later in this chapter, I will talk about some alternatives to sexual intercourse that apply to both men and women—because aging, and change, affect us all.

CHANGES AS WOMEN AGE

Masters and Johnson, the well-known sex researchers and clinicians, have coined the phrase, ''Use it or lose it'' in reference to sexual intercourse. While practice may not make *perfect*, it usually makes for *better* sexual relations. For example, intercourse requires the use of muscles a woman may not otherwise exercise.

The effects of chronic illness may also require you to alter your sexual positions to allow for the comfort of the person who is impaired, and pain may interfere with sexual arousal.

As women age, they may notice a lessening or lack of vaginal lubrication. This commonly occurs after menopause, but may occur at any time. The woman may also notice vaginal itching. (There are many causes for vaginal itching. You should see a physician if this is a problem.) The vagina may be cracked and painful during and after intercourse. This is one of the causes of dyspareunia, or painful intercourse.

Very often the physician will prescribe estrogen replacements to be taken orally, vaginally, or both. In addition to estrogen, the female may need to use a water-soluble lubricant, such as K-Y Jelly. There is also a new product called Lubrin, which is a vaginal suppository that melts immediately to provide lubrication before intercourse. Women should not use petroleum jelly, as it is not water soluble and may allow a freer growth of infectious organisms.

For these and most other changes, communication with your sexual partner is the key. If the problem affects you, it most certainly affects your partner. And if the cause is physical, see your doctor.

WOULD PREGNANCY BE A PROBLEM FOR YOU?

In some cases, younger couples may want to postpone or avoid pregnancy altogether because of the strain and uncertain future of a chronic illness. They must contend with the additional anxiety of a possible unwanted pregnancy.

Chronic illnesses rarely affect fertility. Your reproductive process may be impaired, however, by side effects of your illness such as increased levels of anxiety, reactions to medication, and exhaustion. The likelihood of being surprised by a missed period is higher now because your systems are more unpredictable. I am a believer in planned pregnancies, so I caution you to thoroughly discuss your family plans with your doctor. For your good health, and the health of your children-to-be, plan ahead so you can remain in control of your body.

The topic of birth control needs far more attention than I can give it in this book. All I can say here is that no illness allows you to abdicate your responsibility for your actions as a consenting adult. If an unwanted or unplanned pregnancy would compound your problems, change your strategy.

ALTERNATIVES

" Touch your body and revel in the comfort and pleasure it can bring you. **"**

—SEFRA PITZELE

Below are some alternatives to sexual intercourse. Don't think of these, however, only as "poor seconds." If you or your partner have experienced changes in your sexual relationship, you may find such alternatives more rewarding than your present sexual activities. You may also wish to consider simply adding them to your list of current sexual activities to give yourself some choice when sexual intercourse is not possible or is not desired.

Self-stimulation: Some people feel that since they do not have a regular partner who understands their special problem, they are not entitled to have sex anymore. If the person is newly single after having been married or in a comfortable relationship with another person, the chronic illness or condition may make him feel unworthy of someone else's sexual attention.

The lack of a sexual partner can be ameliorated somewhat by self-stimulation or masturbation. Masturbation is a normal part of every person's sexuality. There should not be guilt associated with masturbation. It is a normal activity which may continue throughout our lives. In addition to manual masturbation, which may be impossible for someone with pain, deformity, or lack of strength in their hands, a vibrator or hand-held massaging shower head may be used to achieve sexual satisfaction. There is even an adaptive long-handled vibrator now available.

Artificial stimulation: Penile shaped devices called dildos can be used by the male to satisfy his partner if he cannot penetrate. Dildos can also be used by a woman if she does not have a partner. Vibrators serve the same purpose. They can also be used to massage the body, to induce relaxation, and to cause arousal before lovemaking.

Oral-genital sex: Some people may be uncomfortable with this alternative, but oral-genital stimulation can provide sexual satisfaction when intercourse isn't possible. The male uses his mouth and tongue to stimulate the woman's sexual organs, and the woman similarly uses her mouth and tongue to stimulate the man's penis. Oral-genital stimulation can be used before sex, during sex, or as sex. Your needs and the needs of your partner determine what approach you take.

Remember that every sexual act need not culminate with a climax. If a person isn't able to have an orgasm for one reason or another, sex can still be gratifying and play an important role in your relationship.

ASKING FOR HELP

If you are concerned about changes in your sexual options, ask your physician for information and help. Be direct and open. Don't allow him or her to dismiss your questions about sex. You are entitled to honest answers. If your doctor suggests you see a sex therapist, you must allow yourself to be completely honest. Don't be shy or embarrased. Be willing to follow his or her suggestions, and you will very likely find that your situation will improve.

For more information, the Arthritis Foundation has issued what I think is one of the most useful pieces of literature on sex and chronic illness. It is called *Arthritis, Living and Loving, Information About Sex*. Many of the suggestions apply to anyone with any type of chronic illness. Some of the suggestions include taking a warm bath or shower before intercourse in order to help relaxation, and timing doses of pain medication so that the maximum effect of the medicine will occur during sex. In addition, the booklet suggests a number of different positions which might be substituted if your usual positions during intercourse have become too painful. I encourage you to read the pamphlet. It's free, specific, and full of alternatives. The addresses for the Arthritis Foundation and other associations which offer assistance are listed in the appendix at the end of this book.

In summary, a chronic illness does not have to mean the end of an active, satisfying sexual relationship. As long as both partners want sex and can communicate what feels good and what hurts, there is no reason why sex in some form should *not* occur. We will always have a need for the warmth, release, and intimacy that sex can bring.

BODYWORK

*T*his chapter covers some of the special physical problems faced by many chronically ill people. I specifically want to talk about joint protection and care of your feet, knees, hips, shoulders, hands, elbows, and back. Finally, I will discuss some special exercise and diet needs and requirements.

An ounce of prevention has always been worth a pound of cure. If your chronic illness, like mine, affects the joints or muscles, learning how to protect them now may save considerable discomfort later in life. This doesn't mean that protection will stop the normal effects of your illness on your body, but you can reduce unnecessary wear and tear and make some of your day-to-day tasks easier to manage.

YOUR FEET

Painful feet will wipe the smile off anyone's face, and there are lots of people who aren't smiling. Foot problems beset an estimated 75–80% of all adults past middle age. Most of us are aware of the more common foot problems. Corns, warts, and callouses top the list, followed closely by toenail problems, bunions, and gout. Rheumatoid arthritis and spurs are also common sources of foot pain.

Feet deserve special care because they carry all the weight of your body. Start by keeping your feet very clean and very dry. After bathing, thoroughly dry each toe and each part of the foot. Inspect your feet often for change. Pain, swelling, sores, or cracking skin should be reported to your doctor immediately. Home remedies are generally not a good idea when a chronic illness is present. Diabetics and people with circulatory problems should be particularly alert to symptoms in their feet.

Whatever your illness, it is important to wear shoes that provide adequate support, and enough room for swollen or deformed feet. A shoe will provide better support if it covers the top of your instep. Most of these lace, or you may prefer Velcro closures if lacing is not possible for you.

The sole should grip the ground well. The shoe should bend exactly where your foot bends. The toe area should be high enough to provide plenty of room for feet that are swollen and sore. You also may have to wear lighter weight shoes. Many of us know the feeling at the end of the day when the extra weight of a heavy shoe seems unbearable.

> **❝ Put your best foot forward, but make sure it's on solid ground. ❞**
>
> ——SEFRA PITZELE

When choosing shoes, remember that your feet need proper ventilation. Leather shoes are preferable because leather "breathes," allowing moisture to escape from your feet. Socks, too, should be made of natural, absorbent materials like cotton or wool. Man-made materials can cause excessive sweating, which can result in fungal infections or sores on your skin.

Women should avoid high heels as much as possible. Walking in this type of shoe thrusts the weight of the body forward onto the front of the foot. If you must wear high heels, keep the following points in mind:

1. A pump is safer than a sling back or backless shoe.
2. Make sure the sole is not slippery.
3. The shoe should be flexible enough to conform to your foot.
4. A heel height of two inches or less is the safest and most comfortable.
5. A wedgie is safer and better for your feet and back than heels.
6. Avoid extremely thin heels.

Finally, if your job requires you to stand a lot, carry with you an extra pair of shoes that have a slightly different cut and alternate during the day.

If you feel pressure in a specific area of your foot or the spot is tender to the touch, ask your physician about the possibility of seeing an *orthotist*. An orthotist has been trained to make inserts and other modifications to shoes. The addition of a specifically formed orthotic inlay may mean the difference between misery and mobility. Some insurance companies cover orthotic devices, so check your coverage ahead of time and remember to get a prescription for the order from your physician.

Some shoes are cut deeper to accommodate inlays. Alsem, E. W. Minor, and Drew all manufacture shoes of this kind. Most local orthopedic foot stores will stock these and other brands that may meet your special needs. Many of the newer tennis shoes have room for inlays and are very comfortable.

People who have badly deformed feet may not find inlays helpful. They may have to wear sandals most of the time to alleviate their foot pain. An orthotist or podiatrist can custom-make a pair of sandals to fit your foot, or you may be able to get custom-made shoes through your commercial orthopedic footwear store.

In addition, a company called Birkenstock sells shoes and sandals that are formed to your own foot. You can order their custom fit footwear by mail. Birkenstock also has retail outlets where shoes can be purchased directly. You can request a catalog or futher information by writing to the company at the address listed in the Finding Help section at the end of this book.

Foot pain can be crippling. We must take the initiative to get the care our feet need. If you need one, insist upon a referral to a specialist. If you are not satisfied, insist upon a *second* referral.

Foot problems serious enough to require surgery can be treated by two kinds of specialists: *Orthopedic surgeons* or *podiatrists*. An orthopedic surgeon is a medical doctor who has completed at least 10 to 12 years of advanced education. He or she performs surgery to preserve or restore the function of the skeletal system and its associated structures in the body.

A podiatrist specializes in the cure of the foot. Some are qualified only to give medical treatment. Others perform surgery, either in a specially equipped room in their offices, or at a hospital. You are the one who ultimately decides whether to see an orthopedic surgeon or a podiatrist. You should consult with your primary care physician when making the decision.

Don't let vanity keep you from wearing the shoes that are best for you. People like you for your personality, not for your shoes.

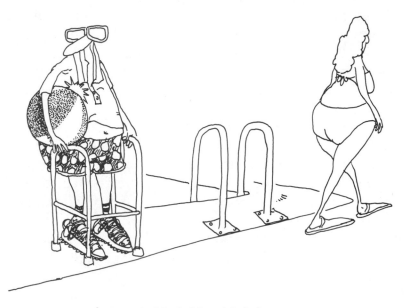

Larry's fake ladder trick fools no one.

KNEES AND HIPS

Knees and hips are also frequently affected by chronic illnesses. Though directed toward those suffering from pain or inflammation in the large joints, most of these suggestions can help everyone.

1. Try to sit in chairs that fit your body. You should have comfortable back support, and when rising, use *both* arms and *both* hips to push yourself up.
2. When getting out of a chair, position one leg slightly in front of the other. Instead of using your fingers for leverage, use your forearms.
3. If you use a cane or walker, be sure it has been measured for you by a professional. One that is too long or too short can cause more problems than it solves.
4. When performing a task at home or on the job, sit whenever possible. Choose a stool or chair that is comfortable and meets your needs.

5. Install grab bars in the tub (or shower) and by the toilet. Consider a raised toilet seat as well.

SHOULDERS AND ELBOWS

Shoulders and elbows can certainly be affected by a chronic illness and they need to be protected as well. Don't get into the habit of leaning on your elbows, which can cause stress to the joint. If you must carry a purse or anything else on your shoulder, try to keep it as light as possible. Generally, as little as possible should be "hung" from your shoulders.

HANDS AND FINGERS

We use our hands more often during the day than any other joints. Like my suggestions for using the large joints, the new and better habits described below could apply even to those not suffering from pain or inflammation now. They can make your everyday life a little easier, and they also may preserve joints which could become damaged with years of abuse. (For names and addresses for some of the items listed below, refer to the appendix on Finding Help at the end of this book.)

1. First and foremost, *never* begin an activity that you can't stop in the middle. What would you do if you were trying to carry something hot, such as a casserole, and your hands did not have the strength to handle the job? Would you be able to put it down or would it slip and break? Plan ahead for contingencies.
2. In general, all movements you make with your hands should be in the direction of the thumb. The inflammation of some chronic illnesses tends to deform the structure of the hand in the direction of the little finger. By making all movements in the direction of the thumb, you may forestall this kind of damage. Numerous everyday actions can be modified to provide the necessary "thumbwise" motion. The three examples listed below can serve as starting points.

■ Learn to use *both* hands when performing a job. If you unscrew a jar lid with your right hand, use your left hand to screw it back on again. This motion makes the fingers of both hands work in the direction of the thumbs.

■ Use the *heel* of your hand whenever possible. When opening a jar lid, washing down a countertop, or smoothing clothing or bedcovers, use the heel or flat of your hand and close your fingers together.

■ Pay attention to how you turn a doorknob. Always use the appropriate hand so that the knob is turned in the direction of your thumb.

3. Try not to pinch your thumb and first finger together. In general, the larger your grasp, the less likely you are to have problems with pain or muscle spasms. Use as large a tool as possible for each job. Here are some examples:

■ Instead of using a thin pen or pencil for writing, create a larger grasp by using a fatter pen, sliding a foam rubber curler over the pen, or getting a pen or pencil adaptor. Even after making this adaptation, you should stop every so often and flex your fingers.

■ Relearn how to cut with a knife, stir with a spoon, hold a hammer, or carry an object. When you wrap your fingers around an object, use as large a grasp as possible. (Remember how you held a knife as a child? Well, back to your old tricks!)

■ When removing a hot item from the oven or stove, either wear insulated mitts and hold the pan underneath with the flat part of your hands, or place it on a heat-proof tray or movable cart. Don't hold it with both hands in a pinched grasp, as it is more likely to slip out of your hands.

4. Never bend your fingers when they could be open and relaxed. If you must lean your head on your hand, place your chin in your palm instead of on your hand with your fingers closed. You can strain your finger joints even when sleeping. Check that you aren't subconsciously tightening your hands into fists as you settle into sleep. If you are, find something soft but resistant to clutch to help you break the habit.

5. Never use your fingers to support any part of your body or to move from a sitting or lying position. Use the largest joints available, such as the heel of your hand or your forearm.

6. Try to routinely move all the joints of your fingers and wrists several times each day. Your doctor or a physical therapist can suggest some exercises, or use your common sense to figure out some for yourself. For example, move your wrist up and down, being careful not to twist it. You should also flex and unflex all your fingers. When doing this exercise, it is best to *bend* inward from the tips of your fingers and

straighten outward from your knuckles. Another exercise is to move your fingers, one at a time, toward the thumb.

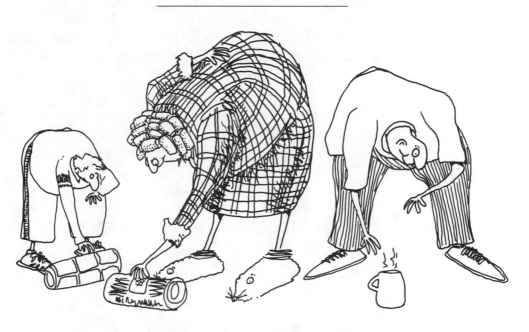

A new way to do range of motion exercies.

7. Make any adaptations in your home or place of work which will make it easier for you to function without causing inconvenience to anyone else. Some of these adaptations could include:

■ Use levers for door handles instead of knobs.

■ Use a wall-mounted jar-opener (such as a Zim) to open jar lids.

■ Enlarge the handles of items which you use daily, such as pens, toothbrushes, carpentry tools, and kitchen utensils. This can be accomplished either by purchasing larger handles or adapting the ones you already have with special dense foam available from a hospital's occupational therapy department or at a local medical supply house.

■ Use electrical instead of mechanical devices. For example, you can imagine how much joint strain is caused by using an old-fashioned, finger-pinch can opener. A can opener which can be operated with one hand is also available.

■ Use a larger sponge and the heel of your hand to exert the most pressure when wiping up or cleaning anything.

8. To move heavy objects, try rolling them or using some kind of lever.

9. If your fingers or thumb bother you each time you open your car door handle, purchase a car door opener which pushes in the handle just as your thumb would.

Finally, learn what is available in the adaptative equipment catalogs and avail yourself of devices you must have to live a more comfortable life. In some cases, insurance will cover items prescribed by a doctor as necessary.

> **" Hands are never too weak to touch something soft or beautiful. "**
>
> ——SEFRA PITZELE

Terry Brady, the Director of Health Education at the Arthritis Foundation of Minnesota, suggests the following clever way to practice hand protection.

My life would be much easier if I lived in France (or Hollywood) where a hug or kiss on the cheek is a socially acceptable greeting, even for strangers. I'd prefer a hug to a handshake anyday. However, I have to face reality here in Middle America, where handshakes are used everywhere—as a form of greeting, to close a business deal, even for congratulations. I'm sure the people attempting to shake my hand are not really trying to torture me, but some days, when my hands hurt, seeing a handshaker coming can make me decidedly unfriendly.

I would like to be an eager handshaker. There's something professional and respectable about extending my hand, but I avoid it. Somehow a grimace would spoil the effect! Over the years I have come up with a number of solutions to the problem, none of them ideal.

My first solution was to avoid any place where someone might be tempted to shake my hand. I gave that up when I realized that about the only place I could go was the bathroom. My next strategy was to seek out the frailest, weakest looking person in the room and settle in next to them. That did not work either. Somehow those people with gorilla grips still found me. I have been tempted to wear my handsplints if I go somewhere that I suspect will have a whole lot of handshaking going on.

Not all of my attempts to minimize the trauma of a handshake have been futile. Sometimes, if I see it coming, I'll try to head off a handshake with a pat on the arm or a shoulder, a greeting without a grip. When both my hands are free, I've had good luck with catching their extended hand between both of mine and giving them a squeeze before they have a chance to squeeze mine. When all else fails, I could do the logical thing and just explain that I'd prefer not to shake hands because it hurts . . . Somehow the logical thing rarely occurs to me. I have seen a button with a sketch of a handshake with a big red X over the top of it—I'm going to ask for a few of those on my Christmas list.

In the meantime, the solution that has worked the best for me is to keep my knuckles out of their grasp. I've discovered the painful part of a handshake for me is when someone squeezes across my knuckles, so when I shake hands I only put my hand in theirs as far back as the first two finger joints. This is still not ideal. In the back of my head I can still hear my father instructing all of his children that "a good firm handshake is the mark of a fair, honest person," but for now this is the best I can do. I'll just have to demonstrate that I am fair and honest without a firm handshake to prove it!

Remember, use good common sense when dealing with joints. If a joint is causing you pain, you can still *use* it if you don't *abuse* it. If a joint is not red or hot, or if the level of pain remains the same day after day, the exercises and joint protection movements may help keep you active and productive.

CHRONIC BACK PAIN

A chronic illness can wreak havoc with your back. However, there are precautions to take to prevent your back from becoming a constant irritation. Start by making a few basic changes in the way you sit, sleep, and lift objects.

Try to always sit on furniture that provides adequate back support. If necessary, prop a pillow behind the small of your back when sitting. When standing, rest one foot on a stool for a while, then switch and stand on the other leg. Your car might also need some modifications to ensure a comfortable posture. Portable back supports can be used in older model cars. Most newer cars have adjustable seats. Further adaptations can be done by a professional; ask your physical therapist for a name or two.

Certain sleeping positions are better for people with back pain. Above all, remember that your back should not be unnaturally positioned during the night. Lying on one side and drawing *both* legs up to your chest is the best position for sleep. Lying on your back and placing a few pillows under your knees also causes less strain on a sore back. Check with your doctor first, however, as some medical conditions prohibit having a pillow under your knees. *Do not* sleep on your stomach with your legs straight. If you have problems sleeping because of severe back pain, check with your doctor for the best position for you.

And *never* lift an object while bending from the waist. Use your knees and hips instead.

If your back gives you more than the usual amount of pain during the day, try to analyze what behavior has caused the pain. If a repetitive task has caused the problem, figure out a way to simplify it. For example, instead of lifting a heavy object from the floor, put it on a dolly and wheel it.

Don't forget hot baths and heating pads! These old-fashioned remedies never fail to provide at least temporary relief. But remember, all the hot baths in the world won't help if you don't learn new habits.

If, in spite of all your efforts at back protection, you continue to have undue pain, see your physician. Besides changing your medication, or perhaps changing the dose of your present one, he may recommend a set of exercises to strengthen your back. Do them conscientiously. They are not difficult, and they will help strengthen your back in the long run.

EXERCISE

Exercise, like religion, is practiced in a wide variety of ways. I do not intend to make an absolute pronouncements about the subject because a particular exercise program might be beneficial for one illness and detrimental to another. Generally, your doctor is the best source of information on the exercise that is most appropriate for you. Nonetheless, one thing is certain: You should exercise as much as you can to keep yourself limber, mobile, and to help your cardiovascular system. Exercise also keeps you from putting undue stress on a particular part of your body.

Even if your illness severely limits your mobility, exercise can help you maintain as much range of motion as possible in each joint. Your doctor or physical therapist can devise a program that takes your limitations into account, yet gradually helps you to go beyond them.

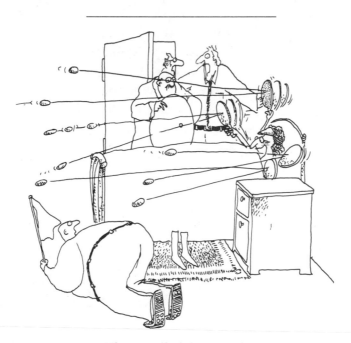

Who prescribed these exercises?

As a rule, exercise falls into the four basic categories listed below.

1. **Active** exercise is performed by the patient, sometimes with the assistance of the therapist.
2. **Passive** exercise involves the physical movement of a part of the body by a therapist.

3. **Assistive** exercise is used when the patient can only move a part of his body to a certain point. The therapist gently assists the patient's movement to increase range.

4. **Resistive** exercise requires the patient to push against an inanimate object to build strength in a specific part of the body.

Exercise should challenge your body without severely straining it. Any pain you feel afterward should be mild and brief. You exercise to increase your body's capabilities, not to punish your body by forcing it to do things it isn't yet capable of.

For those of you who have been active in the past, I should emphasize that chronic illness need not keep you from pursuing your accustomed exercise. On the contrary, it is all the more important to make exercise a habit. Just be sure to check out your exercise program with your doctor. Both your body and mind will benefit from the exercise, and you can take pride in remaining as strong and fit as your physical limitations allow.

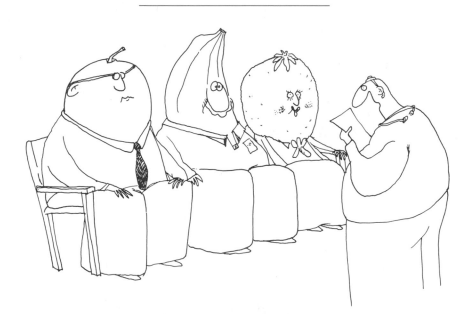

Now let's see, which one of you is on the apple diet?

DIET

Although almost everyone knows the importance of eating a balanced diet to maintain their proper weight, those of us with a chronic illness need to be particularly careful about keeping our weight within the limits recommended by our doctor. If you have any illness that has or will cause impairment of your muscles, joints, or bones, the less weight you carry, the better.

Nonetheless, you may have special problems maintaining your weight as a result of your illness. Pain and exhaustion may make you more sedentary. If you fail to adjust your intake of food accordingly, the pounds will start to accumulate. The stresses of a chronic illness may cause you to nibble out of sheer nervousness, and before long, you wonder where the weight came from.

If you are concerned about your weight and wish to go on a calorie-reduced diet, here are some basic points to keep in mind.

First and most important, *always* check with your physician before going on any kind of diet. You want to be sure you won't be doing anything detrimental to your condition. The same goes for any of the diet books available. Ask your doctor before you apply anything that you have read.

In general, you must make sure your diet is balanced. Don't cut calories at the expense of important nutrients your body requires. Be careful each day to choose food from all four of the basic food groups. In case you have forgotten, here is a list of the four basic groups and the number of daily servings recommended for each.

1. Fruits and vegetables: Four servings daily.
   - One serving may be juice.
   - The average serving is four ounces.
   - Choose carefully because some fruits and vegetables are much higher in calories than others.
2. Milk and milk products: Two servings daily.
   - Use low-fat products.
   - One serving equals one ounce of cheese, eight ounces of yogurt, eight ounces of milk (skim or dry milk powder), or one cup of cottage cheese.
3. Grains and cereals: Four or more servings daily.
   - One serving equals one slice of whole grain bread, one ounce of dry cereal, or one-half cup of cooked cereal, rice, or pasta.

4. Meat and meat substitutes: Two or more servings daily.
   ■ This includes lean meat, poultry and eggs, fish, nuts, and beans.
   ■ Trim all fat and remove skin from chicken or fish. Broil or bake meats and fish instead of frying them.
   ■ One serving equals four tablespoons peanut butter, one cup dried beans, or two eggs.

Next, take a close look at your eating habits. There is more to dieting than simply cutting calories. To be effective, a diet should bring about *permanent* modifications in the way you prepare and eat food. Ask yourself the following questions. Answer them honestly, because they will help you understand your eating habits and possibly change them.

1. Are you aware of how many times a day you eat or drink something?
2. Do you make a real effort to reduce calories in your cooking methods?
3. Have you ever kept a list of all the food you have eaten during a week? Keep a record—you may be very surprised! (Be sure to include all the "just one bites.")
4. Do you eat for solace or when you are bored? Can you find something else to substitute for food?
5. Do you eat during the night or right before bed? Why not try an apple or orange, or a glass of a low calorie drink such as iced tea or no-calorie, no-caffeine soda pop?
6. Do you make an effort to eat *only* when you are hungry? If you have a large appetite or feel hungry frequently, drink a full glass of water or have a salad or piece of fruit 15 minutes before your meal.
7. Do you feel guilty if you cheat on your diet? You may not have evaluated your goals thoroughly enough in relation to your eating habits. Unless your doctor specifically forbids it, everyone is entitled to enjoy some extra calories once in a while. Instead of feeling guilty and adding more stress to your life, adopt realistic attitudes. If you ate more than normal yesterday, eat a little less for the next few days.
8. Have you learned that all food treats need not be high in calories, or that sometimes a small portion is just as satisfying as a large one?
9. Being on the proper diet should be a lifelong commitment. A person *can* alter his caloric intake and permanently lose some weight. Are you really committed to staying as healthy as possible?

Finally, don't be taken in by fad diets that promise miracle weight loss. An effective diet requires a long-term commitment. Remember, weight lost quickly comes back quickly, while weight lost slowly is far more likely to stay off.

On occasion, you may hear about a diet that offers a miracle cure for a chronic illness or condition. "Cure Arthritis with Carrots!" or "Licking Lupus with Alfalfa Pills" are examples of this kind of claim. To the best of my knowledge, there is no proven way to eat your way back to good health. Again, (and this cannot be emphasized too much) talk with your physician about anything you hear about—or you could end up with a more serious problem than you started with.

Let me close by emphasizing that dieting is *not* a punishment. If undertaken with the right attitude, it can be a rewarding, healthful, and enhancing way of life.

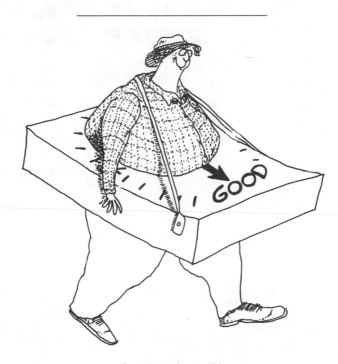

Go where the good is.

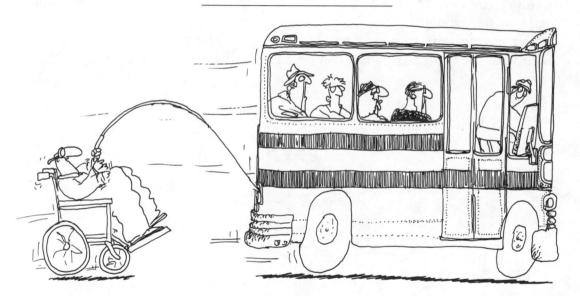

Catching a bus takes on a whole new meaning . . .

ADAPTIVE LIVING STRATEGIES

My life has been separated into two distinct periods: Before Chronic Illness and After Chronic Illness. During the "Before" portion, my life was no different from anyone else's. During the "After" portion, I found that I could live my life as enjoyably as ever, but only with a great deal of advance planning. Believe me, this did not come naturally!

In this chapter, I cover the planning that goes into day-to-day living to help you make a successful adaptation to your new norms. Again, our objective is to achieve the highest quality of near-normal and new-normal lives as possible within the limitations imposed upon us by our particular chronic illness.

After talking with many people who have chronic illnesses, I have concluded that daily routines quickly become some of our largest challenges. Let's look at a scene that is probably familiar to most of us: The struggle to do the family grocery shopping. Our heroine, Susan, takes her responsibility to do the shopping very seriously. Rather than ask for help or delegate it to someone else in the family, she persists in her efforts to carry on with this chore.

Susan used to think nothing of going to the grocery store. She moved quickly and confidently, taking pride in her efficiency and thoroughness. She didn't think twice about spontaneously revising her menus when she came across a good buy, and she often was able to carry two bags at once from the car to the kitchen.

Now that Susan is chronically ill, grocery shopping has changed from a minor task to a major effort. Her pride and sense of responsibility cloud her judgment when she considers whether she is able to handle driving and shopping, and she frequently over-estimates her strength. By the time she eases herself downstairs and out to the car, she is out of breath and starting to hurt. Then, the car door handle won't work, no matter how hard she pushes the button. Finally, the door opens and she gets behind the wheel, but her fingers are so stiff and weak that she can hardly turn the key in the ignition.

At this point, Susan is ready to forget the whole thing and go to bed. She is genuinely worried about her ability to drive the car safely. Still, she remembers that her doctor told her to "challenge herself" to stay active. Besides, the store is only a mile or two away, and the family has to eat. She drives to the store and parks in the regular lot because the handicapped spots have been taken by people who do not have permits. She gets out of the car and walks slowly into the store.

Susan gets a shopping cart and carefully moves along the aisles. Grasping the boxes and cans is hard today. The cans seem so heavy. She drops a few of them and becomes embarrassed and frustrated. She becomes more and more exhausted, and begins to skip some of the less essential items on her list. Soon, she has cut her list down to the bare bones.

When she arrives home, Susan brings in only the perishables and leaves the rest of the groceries in the car. Her children will have to bring them in later. All she can do now is cry. What did she ever do to deserve this illness? It's positively ridiculous! Are things ever going to be better?

Like it or not, much of our self-esteem is wrapped up in those simple, daily things we are accustomed to doing for ourselves and others. Our independence and our role in our families and jobs depends upon doing these chores well. If we take them away, or quit trying to do them, we feel diminished or worthless and we begin descending in a downward spiral of self-pity. How can we have any self-respect, we ask, if we can't even carry our share of the responsibilities?

If we let ourselves go soft and become useless, we'll get exactly what we think we want—a new role: Dependence. If we allow it to happen, we can let our spouse and children and parents and friends put us into a very small box in their minds and hearts—the box they reserve for pity. Sooner or later, we all want more love and respect than that. To get it, we must grow beyond our illness and relearn how to live with risks, anger, discomfort, challenges, and everything else in life.

Susan's efforts were admirable, but she was doing it the hard way. Although that was the way she used to do it, the old ways don't work for her anymore because her body is no longer the same. As long as she continues to ignore the obvious, she will continue to run squarely into her limitations.

Susan and the rest of us have to learn to work smarter, not harder. Our new norms require us to do most tasks a little differently. We will have to do some things much differently, and a few we will have to give up entirely.

I promised you a lot of practical help, and I'm not going to let you down. In this chapter, I share the best ideas I've come across to help you get through the day.

Most of these suggestions are tricks and techniques I learned the hard way as I struggled to regain my independence. Other recommendations come out of the experiences of friends and colleagues who have a chronic condition. I include them for one reason: They work. Use those that suit your situation. Certainly there are many other tips you will discover for yourself in the process.

I challenge you to pick up the pieces of your life that are left and make the most of them. At first, the people around you will probably shower you with support, however small the triumph. After awhile, however, if you've earned it, they will pay you the highest compliment of all and forget about your illness! You know you are making progress when you are treated just like everyone else. Every step toward taking responsibility for yourself is a step away from illness and depression. Planning ahead is the key to this process.

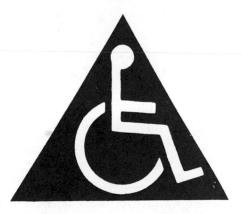

This is the symbol recognized throughout the world for handicapped accessibility and handicapped facilities.

PLAN EVERY DAY TO BE THE BEST DAY YET

With a chronic illness, you must learn to conserve your limited energy. It's more precious now because there is less of it! You can never hope to function independently until it becomes second nature to do your activities in the most efficient, least-tiring way. Each day, in every way you can, look for energy-saving shortcuts.

Effective energy conservation is based on careful planning, and careful planning is based on the elimination of duplicate efforts. Don't do anything twice if you can help it.

My two best rules are:

1. If you decide to do something, do it right the first time so you don't have to do it again.
2. While it is important to approach tasks with a plan in mind, always keep the door open for spontaneous enjoyment along the way.

Let me mentally walk you through a few simple examples to illustrate my point. Before you go to bed, sit down with a piece of paper and a pencil and list your tasks for the next day. (You will soon learn to talk yourself through your errand-running and your work activities.) What *must* be accomplished? What *should* be accomplished? What would be *nice* to get done? Have you allotted time for *yourself*? You may not be able to get everything done, so go into each day with a clear sense of your priorities. You would not want to waste your energy on the unimportant activities at the expense of those that are really important.

Let's say that on a particular Saturday, you have decided to make the bed, wipe up the bathroom, prepare breakfast, clean the kitchen, go to the grocery store, and stop at the bank, the library, and the post office. Not a very formidable list before chronic illness, is it? Let's pull this plan into action without duplicating our efforts.

You can begin your push for efficiency even before you get out of bed. If you can, while still on your back, reach over and pull up the sheets and blankets. Then, position the pillows. It helps if you can use a comforter instead of a bedspread. A comforter weighs less and is therefore easier to maneuver. Then when you get out of bed, all you have to do is give a final flick of the wrist, make a few pulls and tucks, and the bed is made. Before you leave the bedroom, look around. Have you put away everything that needs putting away?

After you have cleaned up and dressed, you can proceed with the second task on your list, wiping up the bathroom. Use large rags which won't tire your hands so quickly. Wipe up frequently so that there is less need for a floor-to-ceiling scrubbing. Get any medicine you need for the day and place it in paper cups or other containers. Finally, check the bathroom to see if you have forgotten anything. So far, so good—and by now, you probably have a sense of how much energy you have for the rest of the day.

Whatever kind of breakfast you eat, always sit down to eat it. Don't eat standing by the counter. You put pressure on your feet, legs, and hips, and you will tire yourself before you have gotten very far into your day. You are also more likely to bolt your food if you eat it standing up. Mealtimes should be enjoyable and relaxing. You should use breakfast to build up your energy level and further collect your thoughts for the day.

Once you have cleaned up the kitchen, you can prepare to do your errands. Gather those articles which you need to take with you. Do you have your keys, coat, and lists handy? Do you have everything you need ready for your stop at the bank? Do you have enough money, your grocery coupons, and library books? Remember, you certainly don't want to waste a trip.

If everything is present and accounted for, think over the route you will take. Use this opportunity to make any last minute changes. If you decide to start with the library, you want to get there before it gets too crowded. How about the bank? That's an easy stop. On Saturdays, you can do your banking at the drive-up window. You don't even need to get out of the car. The post office might be more of a problem. You remember that the post office can be as bad as the library on Saturdays. Visualize what you will have to do when you get there. Do you have the physical stamina to stand in line? You decide the answer to that question is no. You'll try again on Tuesday when it is not so busy. If you are prone to forgetting the sequence of your errands while struggling with the details of getting from here to there, *write it down*.

SHOPPING IS NOT IMPOSSIBLE

Having completed your first errands, you check your list. The grocery store is next. On those occasions when family members are available, I either lasso them into going with me, or I do the shopping and they do the unloading.

Some of the methods I have figured out for saving energy while grocery shopping might help you, too. Because I frequently get tired and have to leave before I buy everything I planned, I make use of what I call a *contingency list*.

The list begins with those items I *must* buy, including toilet paper, milk, eggs, flour, and soap. Then, in order of necessity, I list those items which could be used to prepare two or three decent meals. If I have to leave the store early, I at least have most of the basics and can do some cooking. At the bottom of the list, I put all the extras—things that are nice, but not essential. If all goes well and my energy holds out, I continue through the store and get to cross the extras off my list.

I divide my grocery cart into four areas. In the back of the cart, I place all food items which are already frozen or which need to be frozen. Into another section I put milk, cheese, fruit, and other things that go into the refrigerator. Canned goods go in the third section of my cart. In the last section are the staples for those good old standard recipes, such as the makings for chili, macaroni and cheese, tuna hot dish, meatloaf, and so on. The next page shows how I organize my shopping cart.

I ask the checkout cashier to place each of these sections in separate bags. Because they are organized in the cart, I can unload them approximately the way I want them bagged, making it much easier for the cashier to help me. There are three advantages to this arrangement. First, I find that groceries are less heavy because their weight is more evenly distributed. Secondly, I only need to make *one* trip to the freezer, *one* trip to the refrigerator and *one* trip to the canned goods and staples cupboards. I don't have to sort my groceries and run back and forth to put them away, and thereby save perhaps 15 minutes. Finally, if I don't feel strong enough to unload all the groceries, I can bring in just the perishables and leave the canned goods and dry staples for a family member or neighbor to take care of later. (Incidentally, young children love to make pin money, and this is a great opportunity to make some young friends and get the job done at the same time.)

Planning the grocery store trip in this way allows us a great deal of flexibility. Ideally, we can complete the entire chore, from start to finish. However, if we tire too much, we can still get the necessities. We can usually go back later for the items we had to skip the first time around.

Here are some other tips that can make grocery shopping less tiring and more efficient.

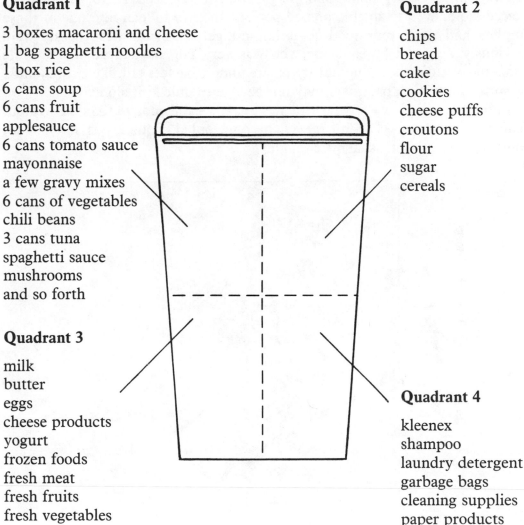

Quadrant I

3 boxes macaroni and cheese
1 bag spaghetti noodles
1 box rice
6 cans soup
6 cans fruit
applesauce
6 cans tomato sauce
mayonnaise
a few gravy mixes
6 cans of vegetables
chili beans
3 cans tuna
spaghetti sauce
mushrooms
and so forth

Quadrant 2

chips
bread
cake
cookies
cheese puffs
croutons
flour
sugar
cereals

Quadrant 3

milk
butter
eggs
cheese products
yogurt
frozen foods
fresh meat
fresh fruits
fresh vegetables

Quadrant 4

kleenex
shampoo
laundry detergent
garbage bags
cleaning supplies
paper products

Store Selection: Choose a store that does not defeat you before you begin. Because you have new needs now, you may have to rethink some old habits and give up a familiar store. When deciding on a store, take into account not only prices and location, but facilities, too, including a bathroom accessible to the handicapped. And be sure you find a store with "user friendly" shopping carts.

Shopping Carts: Some shopping carts are so deep as to be virtually inaccessible, even to an able-bodied person! Just try to lean into one of those jumbos and pack your food so it doesn't get crushed; these beasts were obviously designed by someone who was very tall and stayed home while someone else did the shopping! If you are under five feet tall, have sore joints, or suffer from back pain, you may not be able to unload it alone.

The picture below is my favorite design. It's small enough to move without major effort, the wheels don't seem to become fouled as quickly as others, and, most importantly, it's shallow enough.

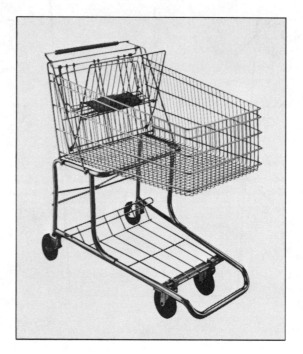

Here's the most "user friendly" shopper cart I've found.

Timing: As with every other daily chore, select the right time to go. Remember that shopping involves going up and down the aisles, a fair amount of brain work, standing and waiting in the checkout line, getting bags into the house, and putting the food away. Use your common sense; shop when you are well-rested and not hungry. Know the layout of the store and plan your list accordingly. Avoid shopping when the store is likely to be most crowded.

Types of Shopping Trips: You may want to try another technique suggested to me by an aquaintance: Reorganize your shopping habits so there are two different types of shopping trips. The first takes care of the milk, bread, eggs, and other weekly perishables that need to be replaced frequently. The second is for staples that can be bought in quantity and stored for future use. Paper products of all kinds, boxed and canned goods, sundries, flour, and sugar are better managed if bought once a month or when you have extra help. If your family members can't help you, hire the paper carrier or the babysitter. Since these boxes and bags don't have to be unloaded right away, you can accommodate your helper's schedule. Also, since you can often buy these items at volume discounts, you can probably break even in spite of paying for some assistance.

Don't Go: When you get right down to the heart of the task, you are really only required to be at the store to write the check and make purchase decisions. If these can be done with a good list and a blank check that can be filled out by a friend or family member, you can still be involved without the exertion. You may even want to explore the possibility of placing phone orders and having at least small orders delivered.

Now, complete your own list and shop and bag this way once or twice to see if you can utilize the ideas. Give yourself a chance to adapt. The whole idea of learning to live with a chronic illness means learning to keep life at a slower, easier, and more convenient pace. Skip the heroics, and learn to make it easier on yourself.

To help make your life a little easier for those days when complete shopping and a complicated dinner aren't possible, at the end of this chapter I have included several quick-to-prepare recipes that are tasty and nourishing. These have become staples at our house and may come in handy when you want a hot meal but your energy level is at a minimum.

Over time, you will develop your own best systems for shopping and meal planning that accommodate your lifestyle and diet.

We could easily spend a great deal of time discussing each activity of a person's day, but I think that you have probably gotten the idea. You know your own schedule, and you alone will have to learn to modify it successfully to suit your own illness. Whatever your day is like, always start it with some kind of a plan like the one we outlined earlier. Plan to make it your best day yet. Even if your day includes only pleasurable activities such as going out for lunch or walking in the park, you should still plan. I do not mean to suggest that a person with a chronic illness cannot be spontaneous or have fun. For everyone's sake, don't turn into a chronic fuss budget and alienate those around you! I am simply stressing that some thought needs to go into the preparation for each task in order to maintain control over the situation. Indeed, you should find that planning makes life much more pleasant because you have enough energy left over to be truly productive and have fun.

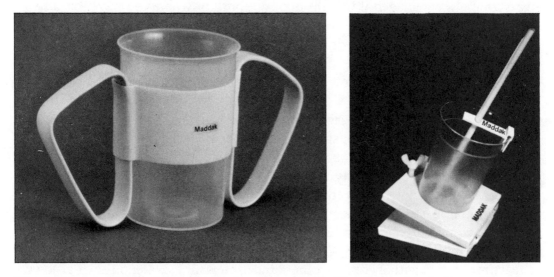

The double handles on this cup make it easier to hold. The tilting glass holder with a straw arrangement may make lifting the glass unnecessary.

GET READY FOR MODIFICATIONS AT HOME

In addition to changes in your routine activities, you may have to modify your physical environment to accommodate your illness. Depending on your situation, you will probably choose one of the following options:

1. Leave everything exactly as it is and manage the best you can.
2. Make discreet, hidden modifications that make your home more comfortable but are not obvious to the casual observer.
3. Make more extensive and obvious changes to your physical surroundings, such as an extra stair railing, grab bars in the bathroom, a seat in the shower stall and so forth, adapted to suit your capabilities.

What you do depends on your physical health and on your emotional willingness to initiate and accept change. In any case, how you organize and run your home will have to undergo periodic reevaluation because of your constantly changing physical needs.

The key is to stop or minimize those motions and activities that cause unnecessary pain or wasted effort. By looking at typical rooms in your house in this context, you will be able to think in a new way about how you do things. We have to think harder to work smarter.

For those of you who have always been well organized, please bear with me—not all of us are. Good organization is the key to convenience in your own home and will contribute to your overall sense of well-being.

THE KITCHEN

Set aside an hour or so to evaluate your kitchen. I did, and it astounded me.

I admit it—I set up my kitchen the way I did because that's the way my mother did it, and it seemed like the natural thing to do at the time. I never really gave it a second thought because it suited my style and my needs at the time. There was no need for other methods or techniques. The only times I even came close to reorganizing were when I had to move something to make room for a new piece of gadgetry! Besides, I was a well woman, so what did it really matter if I carried the roasting pan an extra five steps?

Now, I'm not so casual about how I spend my finite amount of energy each day. These are some of the ways I've changed my kitchen:

Get rid of extras: I went through all the drawers and cabinets and threw away or gave away those items I *never* use. This included four of my five potato peelers and my second toaster, things which I think I kept because I felt unprepared without a "gadget-in-reserve." Now, I have better uses for the room they used to take up. I still don't know how I managed to accumulate 10 wooden spoons.

Organize by activity: Next, I thought about the kinds of work I did in the kitchen and put together all the tools I needed for a particular activity. Remember, we are trying to save our energy and protect ourselves from painful movement. I moved the coffee can, the coffee pot, and the drip filters into the same corner, right by the plug next to the sink. That's an everyday activity at our house and it made a lot more sense to have everything in one place. It may not look quite as chic, but I'm working on camouflaging it with a lovely little plant!

Do you have a baking center? I do now, but it took a little reorganization. I lined a few shoe boxes with foil, and now use them to keep together all of the dry baking ingredients I use, namely the flour, sugar, baking soda and powder, vanilla extract, brown sugar, confectioner's sugar, and carob syrup. Why, for 20 years, did I keep my baking powder in the spice cabinet—and in the back, to boot? Right; probably because that's the way my mother did it and I never gave it a second thought.

I put these baking boxes next to the baking pans I use *and* next to the oven. This has made an incredible difference to me. I've always felt good about baking for my family—it makes me feel as if I'm contributing in a traditional way—and now I feel even better about it because it's not such a painful chore. What a dummy I've been all these years! My only excuse is that conserving my strength and energy was never a problem before, so I didn't have to think about it.

Spices: As long as I was fishing the baking powder out of the spice cabinet anyway, I rearranged the rest of the spices. I put *only* those spices I use daily in front, and relegated to the back the nutmeg and ground tumeric and all the rest of those that I only use for special dishes. Now, I don't care as much if all of the same sized spice tins are lined up together to look neat. When some decorator magazine comes to photograph my beautiful spice rack, I may change it back, but I'm the one who has to use it every day until then.

Pots and pans: My pots and pans will never again be stacked the way they were for many years. Again, all the items I use daily are now in the front, and the waffle iron and roasting pan that I rarely use are in the back. Make it handy for yourself. It didn't make much sense, but I admit that every day for years I lifted my cast iron skillet to get my frying pan just because that's how they were stacked in the cabinet. If you have the space, you may want to hook or hang pots and pans instead of stacking them.

Boxes and canned goods: Arrange your boxed and canned goods according to how you use them. The items you use only occasionally go up above, the ones you use every day stay where they are most accessible. Why keep the box of gelatin at eye level with the pimentos and the kidney beans when it's soup and pancake mix you use daily? Also consider shallow plastic racks that can be attached to cabinet doors for items you use frequently.

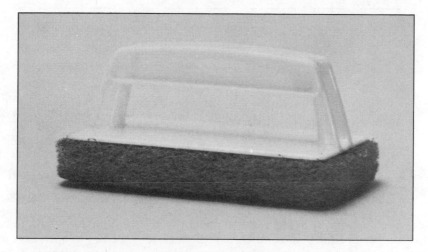

Large rags, sponges, and scrubbers like this one are easier to grip with sore hands. They are less tiring, too.

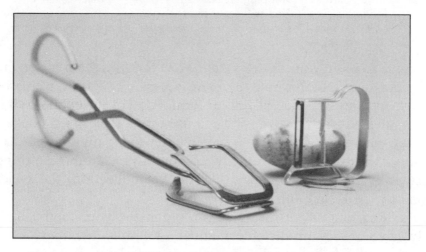

Similarly, tongs and easy-hold peelers can make kitchen work less painful. You will find that you use these more often now, so keep them handy.

Refrigerator: Look in your refrigerator. Do you put heavier items on lower shelves? Are your shelves still in the position they were when you bought the unit? You are not the easy-to-please consumer any longer; make the changes that make it more comfortable for you. Whatever items you use most frequently should be easiest to remove from the refrigerator.

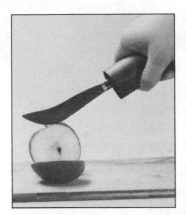

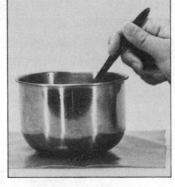

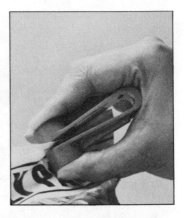

The rocker knife's unique shape helps you get a better "grab" on food. Note the foam roller. A nail or spike through the cutting board helps hold the food in place.

The material under the bowl is Dycem. Because it is a high-friction material, it is ideal for gripping and stopping. It NEVER slips! You will see it in other photos, too.

You don't have to be Hercules to open bags with this slitting device. There is a small blade between the pincers.

Drawers: Look in your drawers, too. Most families seem to use drawers as catch-alls for things that would be more accessible if they were someplace closer to where they were actually used. Remove all of the extra serving spoons and ladles, and put the ones you want to use into a rack or on hooks near the stove. Keep your drawers as neat as possible (try using dividers), because poor organization wastes time and energy. Throw away all those "things" you thought you might need some day (like the key collection, the 2-inch pencil stubs, and the pens that don't write).

Dishes: Rearrange your dishes as you organized your food cabinets. You probably have a very predictable number of family members eating most meals, and they probably use the same glasses and plates. Put these items, plus whatever else you need for a full dinner service, where you can get at them most easily. Put everything else above or below, particularly those heavy serving trays and casserole dishes. You don't need to do battle with them every day.

Light cleaning: Finally, make it easy to keep your kitchen clean by putting the cleaning supplies you need regularly close at hand. You should not have to move eight or more containers of liquid cleaner, at two pounds each, every time you want to do a light cleaning!

Working in the kitchen: Make it a practice to do as much as you can in the kitchen while sitting down. My standard operating procedure now is to work on a few sheets of newspaper covered with wax paper while sitting at my kitchen table. I prepare all my fruits, vegetables, and meat there. I keep my cutting tools and the roll of wax paper in a handy drawer near the table so I can begin the tasks quickly; then, when I'm finished, I just roll up the newspapers and throw everything away. It's simple, fast, and doesn't cost me extra energy.

Don't forget to move your phone or have a longer cord added. Your phone will be more important after your diagnosis, and you should not be wearing yourself out to use it. Incidentally, remember to post near your phone all of the important information related to your illness (See the chapter on Your Health Care Team, pages 105–130).

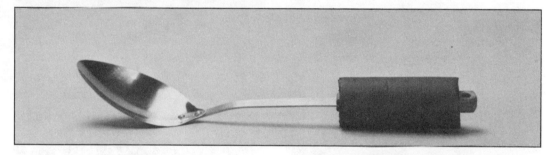

Foam rollers like this make handles larger and easier to grasp.

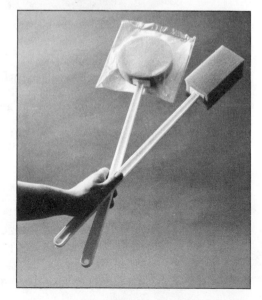

Absorbent foam sponges on handles extend your reach for cleaning projects. Easy to hang and easy to use.

Consider other members of your household: Even though these changes are basically to help you, don't forget the people you live with in the process of reorganizing the kitchen. More than ever before, you are going to depend upon them to help you with certain chores. During those times when you are not feeling well and are unable to prepare meals, they will have to fend for themselves.

Take the time to introduce them to your new system. Ask if they have further suggestions. They have become used to finding certain items in certain places, and it isn't fair to change things without a complete explanation. The next time you try to fix dinner from your bed by giving instructions to a family member, you'll be glad he knows where the utensils are kept.

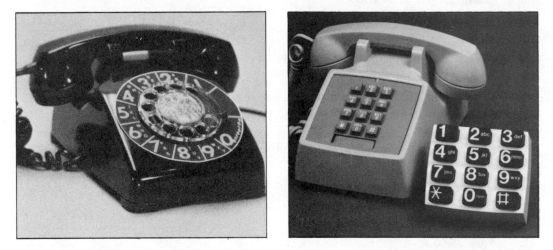

You can make your phone easier to use with these adaptations. The lighted dial helps those with visual impairment, and the enlarged keyboard helps those with reduced muscle coordination. Both are simple plastic attachments and are easily fastened to the phone.

Food: The following tips may be helpful in the preparation and storage of food. Again, the object is to save energy.

1. Unwrap hamburger, flatten it, divide it into meal-sized portions or patties, and place it in a freezer bag. When you need it in a hurry, it will thaw out on the counter in 15–30 minutes.
2. When you feel up to it, brown several batches of hamburger with a few onions and other seasonings. Freeze each batch flat in a freezer bag, and

violà—you now have the fastest ingredients ever for soup, stroganoff, spaghetti, hot dish, and so on. Just combine this starter with fresh ingredients when you need a meal in a hurry.

3. Make a meatloaf ahead of time and freeze it. Use it as an emergency meal when everyone is too busy or too tired to fix anything else.

4. Unwrap, clean, and pack chicken flat for freezing. This way, you can pull out of the bag only what you need, when you need it. Luckily, chicken can even be placed into the oven while still frozen.

5. Wrap and freeze chops, ribs, and steaks individually on a cookie sheet, then bag them together after they are frozen solid.

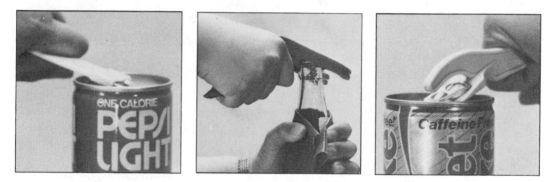

Don't go thirsty! The tab pullers work on the lever principle of physics. The bottle holder is also a bottle opener, as shown. Dycem keeps everything from slipping. Another suggestion: You can hold a can or bottle by closing a drawer on it. By leaning against the drawer, you can hold the item tight until you pry it open.

Accommodative devices for the kitchen: The following accommodative devices will help you deal with specific problems caused by your illness. Since chronic illness does mean forever, I recommend finding solutions to problems as soon as they come up, lest they become an unnecessary drain. I don't like to waste energy and time! Here are some of the devices which have helped make my chores easier.

■ DYCEM: a high-friction material available from an occupational therapist that lets you do many things with one hand. This is my most important aid!

■ non-stick cookware

■ large shaker for powdered sugar and flour

■ sponge mop with pull-up wringer

■ egg slicer

■ Zim jar opener

■ one-handed electric can opener

■ electric knife

■ condiment squeeze dispenser

■ lever to lift can tabs

■ container holder for milk, etc.

■ 2-handled pots and pans

■ garbage bags with handle-ties

■ soap "octopus" with suction cups to keep bowls in place

■ large-handled or two-handled mugs

■ one-handed, suction-cup vegetable scrubber

■ trays or plates for carrying heavy objects (so that they can't slip out of your hands)

■ Lock-Tite step stool with wheels that stop when you step on it

■ pizza cutter: when sharpened, this will also cut meat, bread, or vegetables

■ long-handled dust pan

■ large, soft sponges instead of dish rags

■ sprayer for sink

■ towel or rope tied to refrigerator door for easier opening

■ wooden oven rack slider to push and pull oven racks in and out

■ fire-proof mitts instead of pot holders

■ wooden spaghetti server (which can also be used to turn faucets on and off)

■ foam rollers to enlarge handles of spatulas or stirring spoons

■ long tongs for turning food or picking up small items from floor

■ old foam cushions to kneel on when cleaning

These items are only the beginning of the modifications you will probably make for yourself. If it hurts or wears you out to do it the old way, don't do it like that anymore. Change the way you do it—find a better way. Be resourceful and creative, and you won't have to give in to those kitchen chores that wear you down.

Most of the modifications we have discussed so far have not been obvious to the casual observer who might visit your kitchen. If these are all the adaptations you have to make, count yourself lucky. More obvious modifications include the installation of adaptive appliances, lowering the counter to accommodate a wheelchair, changing cabinet and drawer arrangements and the like.

Remember these basic rules when modifying your kitchen:

1. Strive to simplify.
2. Look for the easiest way to perform the task. Think it through first, and then do it—carefully, please.
3. Whenever possible, sit instead of stand.
4. Keep your sense of humor when the inevitable spills occur.
5. Organize your kitchen according to what you actually need and use most often. If you are not using it regularly, put it up above or down below to make room for a more useful item.
6. Use the lightest weight cooking pots and pans you can; likewise, use lightweight dishes. Perhaps your days of using heavy stoneware are over. So what? Your time is better spent focusing on *real* problems.

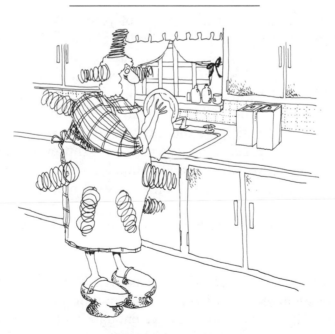

Ethel knows that most accidents occur at home.

YOUR BEDROOM

More than any other room in the house, your bedroom can be your haven. Any flare-up in your condition may force you to spend much more time in your bedroom because of your increased need for rest. Now is the time for a major reorganization that will not have to be repeated unless you have a significant change in your physical needs.

Closets and drawers: Begin with the closets. Both men *and* women have a tendency to hang onto clothes longer than they should, perhaps out of a sense of thrift or wishful thinking that they will someday lose enough weight to wear them. Get tough with yourself and help someone else: Donate everything you honestly don't need or wear, then take a tax deduction. Good for you!

For those clothes you don't wear, but can't bring yourself to throw away—the "maybes"—put a rubber band over the neck of the hangers. Move all of these questionables to one side of the closet, and promise yourself that if the rubber band signifying no use is still there in a year, you will swallow hard and donate those, too.

Organize the "keepers" in the middle of your closet, easily accessible. If you still can't get clothes in and out without fighting with the hangers, find a place for the others, perhaps by packing away all of the out-of-season things. Consider double racks in your closet and plastic modular baskets instead of heavy drawers. Regardless of your type of illness, the day will come when your energy level is low and your joints hurt and the effort of dressing yourself seems to be too much. Anticipate those days and prepare for them now.

The point of this reorganization is to eliminate clutter. Clutter can slow you down and wear you out, physically and mentally. By successfully tackling this chore, you are giving your life additional forward momentum that you need after a diagnosis.

Go through your drawers with the same idea. We all have six to nine pairs of extra underwear, socks, or pantyhose we rarely or never use. Put these in a different drawer or throw them out. Make sure what's left is in a convenient drawer that pulls easily. Handle socks or pantyhose the same way. Get rid of torn pajamas or nightgowns which don't fit anymore.

Getting-into-bed habits: Do you have enough hooks for your pajamas and bathrobe? If not, put some self-affixing hooks on the back of the closet door. It is particularly important with a chronic illness that items are not left on the floor to trip you since the frequency and seriousness of an injury is higher.

Take care to keep the route through the bedroom to the bathroom clear for late-night trips. Incidentally, a nightlight in the bedroom or bathroom can prevent an unnecessary accident along the way. Also, keep a flashlight handy in case of a power failure.

If you like to read in bed, make sure you have adequate light. Since you may have to spend more of your time in bed, invest in a good light that can be easily repositioned and has switches that you are able to use.

If it is at all possible, organize the room so you can turn off all the lights from the bed. Getting out of bed to turn off a wall switch is another needless waste of energy. A bedside lamp arrangement will usually be enough for reading—but don't disconnect the overhead ceiling fixture because that is going to be used more often, too.

By the way, if you have difficulty moving about freely in bed, tricot or satin pajamas *and* sheets will really help.

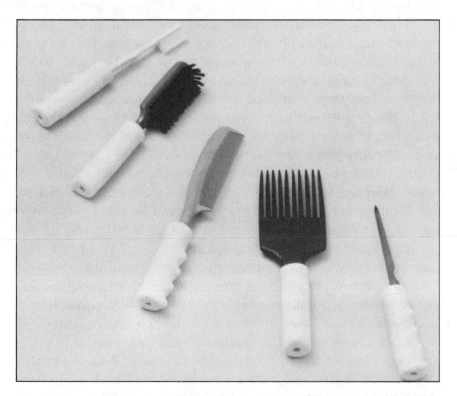

Grooming aids with built-up handles are easier to use. Don't let pain get in the way of looking your best.

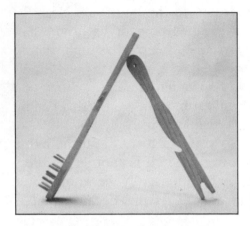

The wooden spaghetti server (left) can also be used to turn faucets on and off. The other device is a nifty wooden "pusher and puller" which can be used with oven racks, among other things.

Furniture: Keep in mind that you are probably going to have more visitors in your bedroom. The practicality of occasionally running your life from the bedroom will quickly outweigh any feelings of modesty or embarrassment. Try to make it as comfortable as possible for someone to visit you by providing a nearby, comfortable chair and an atmosphere of neatness and efficiency. A chair will also be valuable to you as a change of pace. Sitting up for a few hours a day challenges you when you need it without overtaxing your abilities.

A nightstand or TV tray will be invaluable for organizing the essentials: Telephone, a box of tissues, water, medication, reading materials, or projects. If your doctor orders you to rest for a few hours a day (or for any extended period of time), a television with remote controls or a nearby radio can help to pass the time. Handicrafts and hobby tools can also be kept in the drawers of a nightstand. Don't make yourself so comfortable in bed that you don't need or want to get up, but be practical. Life is going to go on without you, so prepare yourself to participate as much as you are able, even if you must temporarily watch from the sidelines during a flare-up of your condition.

Now, check your mattress. Is it comfortable? Firm enough? Since your needs may have changed with the onset of your chronic condition, you may require a change. For the first time in many years, the bedding industry is offering some real options, such as foam mattresses, partial foam beds, air beds, water beds, and adjustable beds. Add extra pillows so you can vary your positions. You may want to substitute your bedspread with a comforter if the spread is too heavy to move easily. Also, since a comforter is usually lighter and more versatile, you can wrap yourself in it and stay warm while sitting up.

You can't kid yourself in your bedroom—you have a chronic illness, and you are going to have to adapt your environment to make yourself comfortable. Remember that the chief goal now is to restore the maximum quality of life as soon as possible. Strive to be as creative and resouceful as you can be to come up with new ways to do old tasks that cause you pain or discomfort. If it hurts, stop feeling sorry for yourself and find another way to do it!

Up to now, I have presented your options as if you were the only one sleeping in the bedroom. Remember, however, to keep the bedroom looking like a bedroom—don't clutter it with so many medicines and paraphernalia that it looks like a hospital room. *Do not* use your illness as an excuse to make someone else's life miserable or uncomfortable. Worse yet, do not use your new needs in the bedroom to fight other battles in your relationship. Love and camaraderie are therapeutic, too, and the bedroom must remain neutral territory. The bedroom should be one place you can always count on to always be comfortable, restful, and restorative.

---

66 By keeping room for the love, there will automatically be room for the patience and understanding you need, too. **99**

——SEFRA PITZELE

THE BATHROOM

The same principles that apply in the other rooms of the house work here, too: Make all the modifications and adaptations you need to make the room safe, convenient, and comfortable. The changes may be obvious or subtle, depending upon your condition. If you have more than one bathroom in your home and you require extensive adaptation, you'll probably only want to make the changes in one of the bathrooms in deference to other family members.

Safety: First, make your bathroom safe. Do you take showers or tub baths? Get the no-skid bath mats you need, and change your bath accessories so that bending and stretching are minimized. Try a shower stool, and use soap ropes or liquid soap in a pump dispenser. Also consider a shower caddy, a hanging basket that hooks over the shower head and keeps soap and shampoo off the floor.

Get rid of *all* glass containers and replace them with plastic. Your joints may not hurt now, and you may feel confident that your muscles will do what you tell them to do today, but sooner or later, you will drop and break something—and face a dangerous situation. You may also need other types of devices, such as grab bars. Don't let vanity stand in the way of safety—if you like, you can paint everything to match your bathroom decor. The grab-bar pictured above looks very contemporary. Finally, make sure the lighting is adequate and all electrical fixtures are safe and easy for you to use.

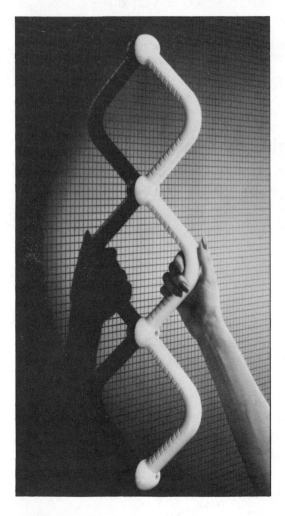

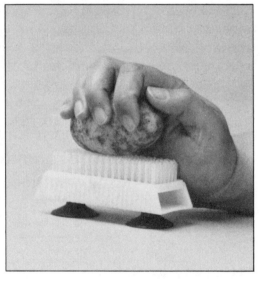

This handle bar for the shower stall is both useful and durable. It looks nice enough to be used discreetly in other areas of the house, too. The suction-cup scrubber is helpful in the kitchen and bathroom alike.

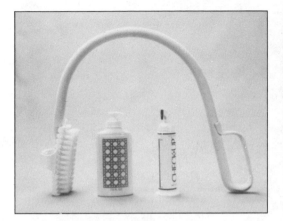

The curved back brush and pump dispensers have helped many people, too.

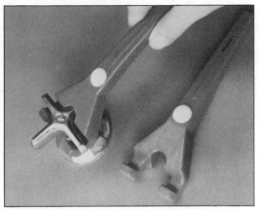

I think these are great: These faucet handles will get you through those days when your joints are stiff or sore.

Convenience: You can eliminate steps by keeping extra towels, soap, tissues, and so forth right in the bathroom, perhaps under the sink or in a drawer. Why do we have to rely on the linen closet down the hall? If you have storage room in your bathroom, use it. If not, stack the towels you'll need that day on the back of the commode.

For those with limited physical ability, a long-handled back brush that curves around the side of your body works beautifully. Incidentally, you may want to trade your wash cloth for a wash mitt or a soft sponge. Sponges are much easier to use when your joints are weak, and they mean less laundry. Toothpaste available in a pump is a boon to the person with weak or sore hand joints. If aerosol cans are too difficult for you to use, try a pump spray or stick.

Keep a roll of paper towels in the bathroom for quick clean ups. A sheet or two can wipe off the sink and keep the rest of the room looking presentable without a lot of effort. Another tip that saves clean up time later: If you occasionally wipe down the glass shower door and the shower or tub with a slightly dampened sheet of fabric softener, soap and water deposits are less likely to build up.

Do as much as you can sitting down, including your personal grooming. This may require that the mirror be lowered or angled downward, and you may have to add a bench or chair. Your illness will probably make you more conscious than ever about looking your best, so you should plan on spending a little more time in front of the mirror.

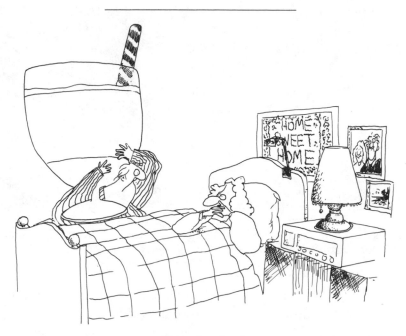

Doctor's orders!

Medications: Just a few words about your medications, which for some reason all seem to end up in the bathroom for storage. Take them all out and line them up on the counter. Open and empty down the commode every one that you and your doctor have tried and ruled out as ineffective for your condition. While you are at it, get rid of the outdated drugs as well.

In addition to helping you comply with your doctor's instructions, you will find that you feel better about yourself each morning if you are not confronted with an array of medicines and pill bottles. Everything you don't use weekly can go into a box in a cabinet or in the linen closet. The Kao-Pectate and Alka-Seltzer will still be there when you need them. Put your daily and weekly medicines out of sight but where you can get to them easily (use a plastic lazy Susan for easy access). If your medications are completely regularized, count them out each week in the morning when you are alert. You can also use a seven-day easy-open pill box that can be carried anywhere with you; it's available at any pharmacy. If you have trouble remembering to take your medicine, devise your own gimmick to remind yourself, such as a medicine bottle turned upside down or a clothespin on the counter.

If you do not have young children around, request *non-childproofed caps* from your pharmacist. Many of us can't manage the "push down and turn" caps. If you wish, you can make this a permanent request so that all your medications come packaged this way.

Think before you move: The secret to making your new bathroom arrangement work is to anticipate your needs and plan your activities. Before you get out of bed in the morning, organize your thoughts. Bring what you need with you into the bathroom so you only make one trip. Keep close at hand the items you need most often. If you plan ahead, you can get into the bathroom, get yourself ready, and be on your way with little or no wasted energy or time. Being able to do this will put you into a better mood and help you get more done, in spite of your finite amount of energy.

Finally, one last word of caution: Without your conscious efforts to the contrary, your bathroom can become the "hospital" room in the house. Like the bedroom, you can keep your bathroom accessible and convenient for everyone by keeping it straightened and presentable.

THE LAUNDRY ROOM

One chore on which you should not hang your personal esteem is your continued ability to perform all the laundry tasks. I don't consider myself a traitor to the principles of motherhood because I taught my family to run the washer or dryer.

I believe that anyone over 11 or 12 years old should be able to wash his or her own laundry. It requires some careful teaching at first, and some gentle reminding later on, but it is definitely worth the effort. Usually a friendly, "The washer is free, does anyone need to use it?" is sufficient.

After teaching them how to use the washer and dryer, the next most important lesson I taught my family was that "doing the wash" meant getting everything back into the bedroom. In spite of their primitive instincts, they are slowly assuming more responsibility, even to the point of separating their own loads, snatching permanent press clothing from the dryer on the fly, and folding it with almost no wrinkles.

They need to understand that by doing their own wash, they are helping themselves and helping you. At our house, when someone is sick—for a short time or a long time—the rest of us pitch in to help. You will be surprised how smart your family actually is. If you trust and believe in them, they will trust and believe in themselves. The fact is you need help, and they are the best around. They might do it differently than you used to do it, but it will get done. Besides, what's the worst that could happen? Perhaps a few clothes ruined? An event like that should not signal the end of your efforts to teach your family. Provide each person with his or her own laundry box or basket, and praise lavishly.

Once your family is ready for the laundry, check your laundry area: Is it ready for your family?

- Is everything in a handy spot?

- Is there easy access to all the appliances?

- Have clotheslines been lowered for those shorter people?

- Does each person have his or her own labeled laundry basket?

- Do you have a reminder board about what items should not be washed together, temperature settings, and a "things to get" list?

- Do you have a place for items which are torn or missing buttons?

- Do you have a good stain remover?

For those of you who live alone, have very small children, or for some other reason do not have the help you need, I have a few suggestions.

Do everything you can to streamline and organize your laundry chores. This may mean you get a few more baskets or wash more frequently to reduce the number of heavy loads. Or change the times you do the wash to match the time when you have enough energy. The list above will help you put your laundry room in order, too. If you do your laundry in the basement, you can conserve energy by keeping a folding lawn chair, a book or television, and, if possible, a phone nearby. In this way, you can stay downstairs if you have to until the chore is complete.

If all else fails, look elsewhere for another pair of hands to help you. There are no magic wands or incantations to get your laundry done for free, so be prepared to pay someone else to do it. There are a broad range of services that can solve at least parts of the problem if you care to shop for them. A professional dry cleaner and laundering service should be easy to find. It may not be as easy to find one who picks up and delivers, but they are out there.

Other cleaning services are available in the yellow pages of your phone book.

If you have a reliable babysitter, she may be willing to help you for a few extra dollars. If you belong to a condominium association or social club, you may be able to find someone with similar needs or a similar schedule who you can help in return for their assistance. Teenagers are always looking for ways to make money.

No matter how you get your clothes clean, there will still be some ironing. To protect your joints, get one of the newer lightweight irons or a small press. I suggest you do your ironing in the bedroom or some other place where you can sit down. Indulge yourself with a favorite TV program or record. Of course, I consider the required care much more seriously now when I buy clothes, so I am doing less and less ironing. Other members of your family can be taught to iron, too!

YARD WORK

If you're like me, working outside is a treat. I urge you to fight hard to keep it a part of your routine. You have to use your common sense, though.

There is a tendency to overdo yard work. Because there is usually a definite beginning and end to each task, many people are reluctant to quit before they have finished the job. "After all," they reason, "the yard will look funny if I cut only half the grass, even though that's all the energy I have." Yard work can become very difficult if you take it too seriously.

Learn to recognize those tasks that are too large for you to handle. Admitting when you have reached your limits is a sign of maturity and successful adaptation, not weakness. If you love to garden, but can no longer tackle a large one, how about a series of window boxes?

Check with the neighborhood children or the local youth employment services. My experience has been that there are plenty of young people ready, willing, and able to help out for a very reasonable charge. As suggested before, perhaps, you can barter rather than pay. "You mow my lawn, I'll mend your clothes."

Do what you can. At the back of this book, I have identified some of the catalogs that feature adaptive yard equipment such as two-handled shovels and roller snow shovels. Even if you do no more than pick up the litter with a stick-and-nail spear, you will get a feeling of genuine satisfaction. A sense of self worth is critical to your happiness. If the chore you want to perform is substantial but you want to tackle it anyway, you may want to plan your day around it and conserve your energy accordingly.

Inside or outside, remember the key to successful adaptation is the conservation of energy. If you conserve your energy as well as you can, you will have the strength and courage to improve your quality of life.

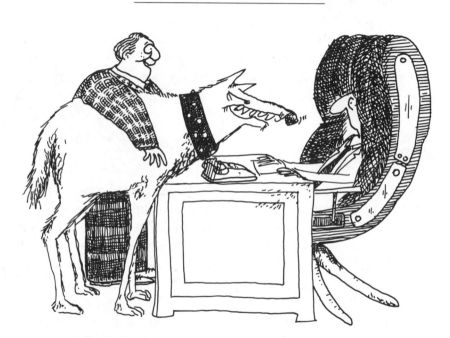

How NOT to discuss your condition with your employer.

MODIFICATIONS AT WORK

Your rights as an employee: If you work outside your home, you may be able to continue working at your regular job if your illness is not immediately debilitating. Holding on to your job means you will have a vastly improved chance of maintaining your lifestyle, your positive mental health, and your self-esteem. Whether or not you continue to work depends on how well you feel, your attitude, and your employer.

Imagine the fate of Renee
Who broke dishes three times in one day.
She fussed and she fumed
As she swept up the room
And wished her disease would go 'way.

——SEFRA PITZELE

Termination laws: In most states in this country, it is illegal for an employer to fire a person because of an illness or disability. Personal issues related to your illness, however, such as tardiness, productivity, attitude, or work motivation *could* cause your termination. In some instances, a mutually acceptable job transfer is required to accommodate the illness.

Communication with your employer: As soon as you are fully aware of the extent of your illness as it affects your work productivity, talk to your employer and, if possible, write out, sign, and date the agreements you jointly reach. *Don't,* however, under any circumstances, sign anything relating to workers' compensation benefits until after you have consulted an attorney. Clear and frequent communication between you and your employer will assure that your options are left open as long as possible and your interests are protected.

Your employer needs to know if you can continue doing your job effectively. If you can't, what specific restrictions and limitations do you have? Are you going to have periodic flare-ups and miss some work? Do you need special modifications at your work site? Will you need restbreaks during the workday? Explain what you expect to happen and what your needs are to the best of your ability. Give your employer permission to call your physician for verification and clarification of what you are telling him.

During these early conversations, it is important to avoid an adversarial relationship. Employees fearful of losing their benefits and employers fearful of being taken advantage of are equally prone to overreact. Keep in mind that a good employee—like you—is difficult and expensive to replace. Your employer is more likely to fight to keep you on the job, rather than fight to get rid of you.

Changes at your work site: In some cases, all that will be required to stay in the same job will be a physical change in your work area or hours. For example, a job done standing can often be modified so it can be done while sitting. Furniture could be moved to save you a few steps. Most employers already have bathroom facilities that accommodate the handicapped; if yours doesn't, the problem is easily solved with some door modifications and some grab bars. If one looks hard enough, there is federal money available to pay for these modifications, but it takes patience to find it. Also, the local trade or vocational school will often come in and make the modifications just for the experience if the company pays for the materials.

Often the only change required at the outset will be a little more rest during the day. Your employer might be willing to break your hour lunch into three segments: 15 minutes to rest, 30 minutes to eat and another 15 minutes to rest.

Rest: Make sure you really rest. Sitting down and having a cup of coffee, alone or with friends, takes the strain off your mind, but not off your body. You must try to rest completely for a short time to restore your strength. These short periods of rest will make the difference in your ability to survive your job. Most work places have some sort of employee lounge. Find an old easy chair or sofa you can use; if one is not available, see about getting one in, even if you have to buy it yourself secondhand.

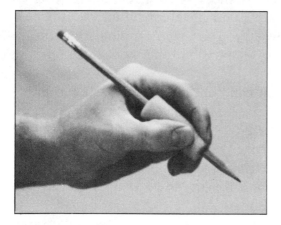

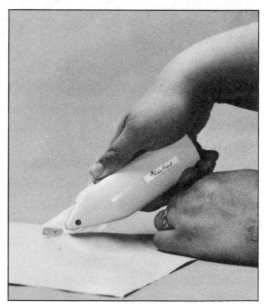

The foam on this pencil stems writer's cramp.

Believe it nor not, these electric scissors actually cut things!

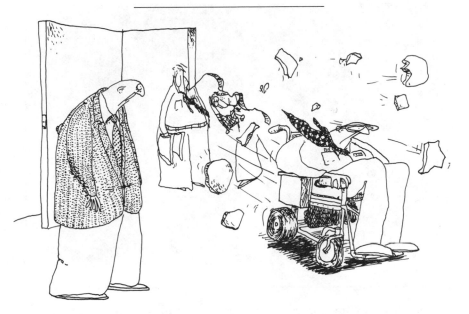

Horace makes another request for wider doorways.

Relationships with your colleagues: Don't make your need for rest a secret or private affair, but don't cause hard feelings by advertising any special treatment you receive. After the initial awkward feelings have passed, most of your friends and colleagues at work will accept the situation as normal. Most of them have probably had some limited exposure to chronic illness of one kind or another, although it may have been a negative experience for them at the time. They may begin to ask you questions about your illness. Try to be simple and honest with them, making the point that chronic illness can vary from day to day and that you're not receiving privileged treatment or just being lazy. You may want to keep some informational brochures handy for those who are really interested. Don't wear your illness on your sleeve—people still don't enjoy hearing every last detail about someone else's troubles—but let them know that some days are better than others. They will be proud of you when they see that you are working hard and carrying your fair share even with a new medical problem. Be confident that the people who are your friends will remain your friends.

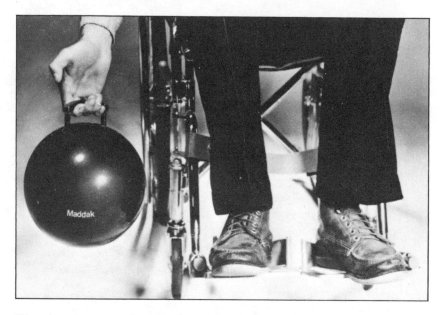

There's no excuse for not participating as well as you can! This is a
bowling ball with a retractable handle.

Keep your office acquaintances and friendships as active as you want them
to be. If you are on a bowling team, for example, go as often as you can and
participate at whatever level you feel comfortable. You will become expert at
politely letting people know how you feel with just a few words that do not
bring undue attention to yourself or spoil the fun for others. Comments like,
"I'm just going to be scorekeeper tonight," or "I think I'll sit this one out,"
gently but firmly let you steer your own course.

The weekly tennis game or the morning jogging may have to be changed to
a lunch date or a walk instead, but the people are still the same. Do the best
you can to let your friends see that you are attempting to live as "normal" a life
as you can. And since you are not feeling sorry for yourself, they shouldn't feel
uncomfortable either.

You are not going to win with everyone. Some people are not going to be
able to accept the changes that are coming over you, and they will drift away.
But others will drift in to replace them, people who understand and are willing
to accept you as you are. The longer you have been at your job, the deeper the
friendships and the commitments will be.

If you are thinking of leaving: The day will come when you may have to or want to leave your job. Carefully investigate your options and their implications, however, before finalizing that decision. This is especially important in relation to medical or retirement benefits. If you are being threatened with termination because of your condition, call an attorney for professional legal advice. Remember that it is illegal and discriminatory for you to be fired for your illness or disability. Such action exposes the company to legal remedies executed by you to protect your rights.

Many companies offer short-term disability and other benefits, and you must remember that you are entitled to those benefits. You may need to be off work for a short time during a flare-up or during a period of rehabilitation, but do not allow yourself to be convinced that you cannot ever do the job again. Perhaps if you cannot do *that job*, there are similar jobs that would be more suitable elsewhere in the organization. Most states have information readily available regarding your rights. After you've left, it will be too late—you *must* be your own advocate *before you leave*.

This Maddak walker is one of the best I've found. It's adjustable, features a sling-type seat that lifts up out of the way, and is lightweight. The hand grips are adjustable and contoured at the front to prevent your hand from sliding forward.

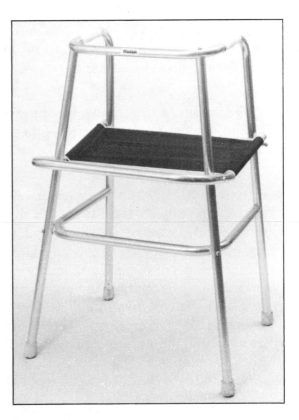

PHYSICAL THERAPY

A physical therapist has been trained to help a person regain strength, movement, coordination, range of motion, and endurance, and perhaps to delay some deformities. Physical therapy must be initiated by a physician's order. An individualized plan will be developed for each patient. A wide variety of treatment modalities, from heat to nerve stimulation. A physical therapist is a crucial member of the health care team.

OCCUPATIONAL THERAPY

If your physical limitations require you to develop new living and working habits, you may want to consider assistance from an occupational therapist.

An occupational therapist has been specially trained to help people with a medical condition (recent or longstanding) achieve maximum functioning in the workplace and at home.

Patients are usually referred to an occupational therapist by their physician. In many cases it is up to us to ask our doctor for this kind of help. Most doctors don't think of asking questions such as:

"Do you have any trouble brushing your teeth?"
"Can you get your shoes tied without any problem?"
"Are you able to drive easily?"

If you don't tell him, he'll never know and you'll never get the help you need. Occupational therapists are one of the greatest resources for people with chronic conditions and are often underutilized by patients and their physicians.

On the first visit, you can generally expect an occupational therapist to read your doctor's prescription and any medical records pertinent to your specific case. He or she will then interview you to evaluate your problems and needs.

Finally, the therapist will work with you for a short while to determine what your limitations are. He or she will devise a personalized program based on those limitations.

After the first visit, appointments are generally scheduled every day or twice a day for hospital inpatients, and one or more times a week for outpatients.

As therapy progresses, you will gradually learn how to cope with the situations that were a problem before. Some people, for example, find that as a result of their illness they can no longer use standard bathrooms. Many occupational therapy areas have models of bathrooms equipped with raised toilets, grab bars, and other modifications that allow greater accessibility. The therapist instructs and demonstrates how to use the bathroom independently. Practice continues until the patient is fully comfortable with the equipment and with other techniques for adjusting to his physical limitations.

In addition, most occupational therapy clinics have a full or modified kitchen area which is built to accommodate wheelchaired as well as ambulatory patients. Whether or not you are a homemaker is irrelevant; most of you have kitchens and want to be able to use them.

Occupational therapists are also concerned with fine motor coordination. Washing, grooming, and dressing are everyday activities which make use of fine motor coordination. A therapist can often suggest an accommodative aid to help people who have difficulty with smaller, more concentrated movements. For example, I had difficulty cutting my fingernails and using a scissors because my hands cramp so badly. The occupational therapist ordered a nail clipper with a special grip and a pair of spring-action scissors for me. These may seem minor items, but they made a major difference in my everyday life. The once-routine task of cutting my nails became routine again.

Some occupational therapists take further training and specialize in working with hands and joints. They may share office space with a hand surgeon and work with that surgeon's patients. If you have particular problems with your hands, you may want to talk to your physician about seeing a hand specialist. In general, hand therapists perform three functions: They create splints and other devices to prevent deformity or to protect the joints, they rehabilitate a hand or finger after surgery or injury, and they work with patients to develop dexterity and strength.

Whether you choose an occupational therapist or a hand surgeon, keep in mind that you will need a doctor's referral and pre-scheduled appointment before you can see either. By all means, take advantage of this invaluable resource. Occupational therapists and hand therapists can help you through the changes that are inevitable with any chronic illness.

ADAPTIVE AIDS FOR AUTOMOBILES

In some cases you will have to adapt your car for your comfort or to accommodate changes in your body caused by illness.

In most large towns, there is a company that can install various adaptive devices for your car. These include knobs for the steering wheel, specially formed back supports, special brake or gas pedals, hand controls, and fully outfitted vans with hydraulic lifts.

In addition, other helpful devices can be purchased through catalogs. These include a car door opener (if your car has a push button door), an enlarged key ring (for ease in unlocking and starting the car) and a tool which can be used to reach across the car and unlock the other door from the inside. If you are the passenger instead of the driver, consider a front seat that swivels out toward the door and a seat that reclines.

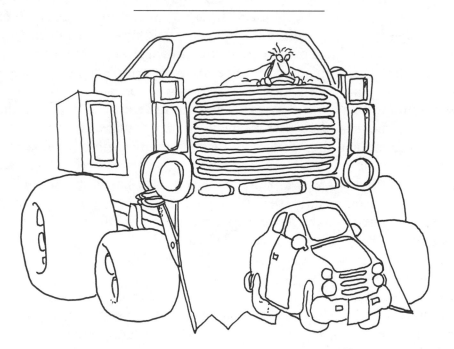

Frank enforces the "Handicapped Parking Only" regulations in his city.

If you are purchasing a car, you should also be aware of some options which can make your car comfortable instead of a torture chamber.

1. Lift-up door handles rather than push-button openers.
2. A tilting steering wheel so you can get in and out of the seat easily.
3. If strength is a problem, choose a non-friction upholstery, such as vinyl or leather. Velour and fabric do not allow easy slide-ability. If you do choose fabric, spray it immediately with a fabric protector so spills are easier to clean.
4. Easily adjustable seats. If knobs or handles are a problem for you, choose a car with levers. Seats should adjust several ways and support your back well.
5. Power windows and door locks if possible.
6. An automatic trunk-release to save getting in and out of the car so many extra times.
7. Adequate trunk space for packages or a wheelchair, if necessary. It is easier to lean into the trunk than to crawl into the car to get groceries.

While I am on the topic of cars, this would be a good time to mention *handicapped parking permits.* In most states information and an application form may be acquired from the Department of Motor Vehicles or from your state handicapped advocacy office. Your doctor will have to fill out part of your application. Once you have a permit, it usually need not be renewed. Use it wisely; it is intended to make our lives just a little easier.

Just a word about license plates which signify the driver is handicapped. This is strictly a personal choice, but since the handicapped permit allows parking in a designated zone anyway, you may want to reconsider getting license plates designating a handicapped driver. I have heard more than one story about drivers with handicapped plates being taken advantage of, especially if you have car trouble on the road. Sometimes it is better not to announce that there is a disabled person in the car.

AIDS FOR THE AUTOMOBILE

Below are places to write for information about adaptive devices for your car, and sources of air and bus travel information.

Amigo Sales, Inc.
6693 Dixie Highway
Bridgeport, MI 48603

Care Chair Systems, Inc.
5602 Elmwood Avenue
Indianapolis, IN 46203

Rehabilitation Equipment and Supply
1823 West Moss Avenue
Peoria, IL 61606

Southeastern Mobility Co., Inc.
8236 Middlebrook Pike
Knoxville, TN 37919

American Automobile Association
1712 G. Street N.W.
Washington, D.C. 20015
(Request a free list of automobile hand-control manufacturers)

MORE ABOUT TRANSPORTATION

Access Travel: A Guide to Accessibility of Airport Terminals
U.S. General Services Administration
Washington, D.C. 20405

Air Traveler's Fly Rights
Office of Consumer Affairs
Civil Aeronautics Board
Washington, D.C. 20428

Air Travel for the Handicapped
TWA
605 Third Avenue
New York, NY 10016

Helping Hand Service for the Handicapped
Greyhound Lines
Greyhound Towers
Phoenix, AZ 85077

QUICK AND EASY RECIPES

In the last two editions I promised and printed several recipes, which I called "survival recipes." They were easy and quick.

Apparently more people than I was aware of are concerned about their hearts and the build-up of cholesterol. So this time with the permission of the American Heart Association Cookbook's publisher, David McKay Company, New York, I am instead printing several "heart-safe" recipes. They taste wonderful, and none of them are hard to prepare.

TUNA QUICHE IN A RICE CRUST

Ingredients

¾ cup dry brown rice
2 cups water
3 eggs (6 egg whites or egg substitute equivalent to 3 eggs)
1 teaspoon dill
1 10-ounce can water-packed tuna
1 tablespoon lemon juice

1 medium onion, chopped
1 tablespoon parsley, chopped
1 cup skim milk
⅓ cup sharp cheddar cheese, grated
10 mushrooms, sliced
½ cup green pepper, chopped

Directions

1. Cook rice in water, till tender, about 40 to 50 minutes. Mix with 1 beaten egg and dill. Press into 9″-pie pan, forming a crust. Bake at 350°F in oven for 8 minutes. Remove.

2. Mix tuna with lemon juice, onion, and parsley.

3. Mix 2 remaining eggs with milk and cheddar cheese.

4. Assemble quiche by placing mushrooms on the bottom of the crust. Add the tuna mixture and sprinkle with chopped pepper.

5. Finally, pour egg and milk and cheese mixture to cover. Bake at 425°F for 10 minutes. Reduce heat to 350° and bake for 30 additional minutes. Quiche is done when center is firm.

Yield: 8 servings
Approx. cal/serv.: 175

CHICKEN À LA KING

Ingredients

3 tablespoons oil
4 tablespoons flour
　freshly ground black pepper
3 cups chicken stock
⅓ cup nonfat dry milk
½ pound sliced mushrooms

¼ cup diced green pepper
¼ cup chopped pimiento
2 cups cooked chicken
4 tablespoons sherry
1 tablespoon chopped parsley

Directions

1. Heat oil in a saucepan, add flour, and cook briefly, stirring. Pour in chicken stock, stirring constantly until thick and smooth. Season and stir in nonfat dry milk. Cook 1 minute.

2. Sauté sliced mushrooms and add to sauce, along with chicken, green pepper, and pimiento. Heat through, then add sherry. Adjust seasoning, and garnish with parsley. Serve with rice.

Yield: 6 servings (about 1 quart)
Approx. cal/serv.: 1 cup = 205 (or 305 with ½ cup rice)

CHICKEN CURRY—IN A HURRY

Leftover roast or boiled chicken can come to no better end than in this zesty dish of Eastern origin.

Ingredients

2 cups cooked diced chicken or turkey
½ pound thinly sliced fresh mushrooms
1 tablespoon oil or margarine
⅓ cup chopped onion
3 tablespoons flour

1 cup chicken broth
1½ teaspoons curry powder
1 cup finely chopped apple
¼ cup chopped parsley
¾ cup skim milk
1 cup water

Directions

1. In a large skillet, sauté chicken, mushrooms, and onions in oil until chicken is lightly browned on all sides.

2. Stir in flour, broth, and curry powder. Add apple and parsley; then pour in milk and water. Simmer, stirring constantly, for 3 minutes or until apple pieces are tender-crisp.

3. Serve over rice.

Yield: 4–6 servings
Approx. cal/serv.:235 (or 335 with ½ cup rice)

BEAN SPROUT TUNA CHOW MEIN

Ingredients

1 cup chicken broth
1 tablespoon soy sauce
  freshly ground black pepper
2 tablespoons cornstarch
6 stalks celery, cut diagonally
2 medium onions, slivered
1 6-ounce can bamboo shoots, drained

1 4-ounce can mushrooms, drained, or 4 ounces sliced fresh mushrooms
2 cups freshly grown bean sprouts or 1 can bean sprouts, drained
2 tablespoons oil
1 7-ounce can water-packed tuna, drained

Directions

1. Mix chicken broth, soy sauce, and pepper. Stir in cornstarch until dissolved.

2. Slice celery diagonally ⅛ inch thick. Slice onions in very thin slices or slivers. Cut mushrooms in slices.

3. Heat oil in frying pan or wok over highest heat. When hot, toss in celery and onion; stir-fry 1 minute. Add bamboo shoots, mushrooms, and bean sprouts.

4. Stir broth mixture and add to vegetables. Stir and cook just until sauce is thickened. Add tuna and stir until hot and sauce is clear.

5. Serve immediately over fluffy rice.

Yield: 4 servings
Approx. cal/serv.: 220

LAZY BEEF CASSEROLE

A delicious gravy forms during the cooking of this very easy and tender beef dish.

Ingredients

1 pound lean beef chuck, cut into
   1½-inch cubes
½ cup red wine
1 10½-ounce can consommé, undiluted

¼ teaspoon rosemary
   freshly ground pepper
1 medium onion, chopped
¼ cup fine dry bread crumbs
¼ cup all-purpose flour

Directions

1. Put meat in a casserole with the wine, consommé, pepper, rosemary, and onion. Mix flour and bread crumbs and stir into the liquid.

2. Cover and bake at 300°F., about 3 hours. (Or, a lower temperature and longer cooking time may be used if it is more convenient.)

3. Serve with rice or noodles.

Yield: 4 servings
Approx. cal/serv.: 350 (or 450 with ½ cup rice or pasta)

By popular demand, even though they are not from the American Heart Association Cookbook, many folks have expressed their pleasure at the ease and taste of the following recipes.

THE EASIEST LASAGNA EVER

Ingredients

1 to 1½ pounds lean ground beef
4 cups prepared spaghetti sauce
1 pound grated mozzarella cheese for
   topping (if you grate it yourself, you
   get more)

1 box lasagna noodles
   Boiling water

Directions

1. Brown hamburger and drain.

2. Add spaghetti sauce (we love Prego).

3. Preheat oven to 350°F.

4. Spread a little of the meat and sauce on the bottom of a 9″ x 12″ pan.

5. Layer raw noodles in whichever way they best fit.

6. Add spaghetti sauce with meat, then cheese, then noodles.

7. End with sauce and some cheese, holding out a little of the cheese end.

8. Pour boiling water right into the edges of the pan to within ½″ of top.

9. Cover *tightly* with aluminum foil and bake for 40 minutes.

10. Now, uncover and bake for 20 more minutes.

11. Bake 10 minutes more with a little more cheese sprinkled on top.

12. Let set for 10 minutes before slicing.

Total preparation time: 15 minutes
Total cooking and holding time (while you are resting or doing something else):
1 hour, 20 minutes

WILD RICE HAMBURGER CASSEROLE

Ingredients

1 small box Uncle Ben's Wild and Regular rice mix (not instant)

1 to 1¼ pounds lean ground beef
1 can cream-of-anything soup

Directions

1. Cook wild rice according to directions.

2. While rice is cooking, brown, season, and drain beef.

3. Add the can of soup, undiluted.

4. Mix with rice and serve immediately.

Total preparation time: 20 minutes

TURKEY OR CHICKEN TETRAZZINI

Ingredients

¼ cup margarine
¼ cup flour
1 cup chicken broth
1 cup whipping cream
2 tablespoons sherry, if desired

1 7-ounce box of spaghetti, cooked and drained
2 cups of diced or slivered chicken or turkey, cooked
1 6-ounce can of mushrooms, if desired
½ cup grated parmesan cheese

Directions

1. Preheat oven to 350°F.

2. Cook spaghetti according to directions.

3. Blend margarine and flour; cook on low heat.

4. Stir in the cream and broth, heating until it boils for at least 1 minute. Keep stirring during this time.

5. Add the chicken or turkey and toss all together.

6. Pour into a lightly greased 9″ x 12″ casserole dish.

7. Sprinkle the parmesan cheese on the top.

8. Bake about 20 minutes.

Total preparation time: 20 minutes
Total baking time: 20 minutes

THE EASIEST CHILI EVER

Ingredients

2 pounds ground beef
2 large cans stewed tomatoes
2 cans tomato soup

Chili powder
1 can kidney beans

Directions

1. Brown hamburger and drain.

2. Add stewed tomatoes, undiluted tomato soup, and beans.

3. Add whatever seasonings and the amount of chili powder you like.

4. Simmer until done, anytime from 30 minutes to 2 hours.

5. For a special treat, add colby cheese and grated onion on top!

ENGLISH MUFFIN PIZZAS

Ingredients

Enough English muffins for your family
Whatever meat and cheese you like to use

Pizza sauce or leftover seasoned spaghetti sauce

Directions

1. Split the muffins.

2. Spread with the sauce.

3. Cover with the meat and cheese.

4. Broil for a minute or two.

Total preparation time: 5 to 10 minutes

BEEF STROGANOFF

Ingredients

  1 pound trimmed, thinly sliced beef   1 can condensed beef broth
  ¼ cup margarine or butter   1 cup sour cream
  6 ounce can mushrooms   2½ tablespoons flour
  ½ cup chopped onions

Directions

1. Trim and thinly slice beef.

2. Brown meat in the margarine or butter.

3. Add the mushrooms, drained.

4. Add the chopped onion.

5. Simmer all together very gently for 4 to 5 minutes.

6. Add the condensed beef broth. Heat.

7. Blend the sour cream with the flour.

8. Simmer very gently until it thickens.

9. Season to taste.

10. Serve over noodles or rice, or use as a main course in a baked potato.

Total preparation time: 20 minutes

PRACTICAL MATTERS

*T*his final chapter addresses a few practical matters which at some time or another will probably affect all of us who have a chronic illness or medical condition. I've included information on your rights as a patient, different types of health insurance, and sources of financial and medical assistance.

Every person I meet has a new idea or worthwhile suggestion I want to pass along. As each of us continues to grow, I just hope we all remember our own early struggles with change so we can reach out and help others.

I would welcome your suggestions and ideas. Please take a few minutes to complete the Reader Survey at the back of the book and drop me a note in the process. We're all in the same boat, so let's start rowing!

WHAT DO I DO WHEN I MEET A PERSON IN A WHEELCHAIR?

Meeting someone in a wheelchair should not be an awkward situation; however, many people are unsure how to act, which can create some embarrassing moments. The rehab staff at Schoitz Medical Center has prepared this informational guide of wheelchair etiquette to help prepare people for encounters they may have with wheelchair users.

1. *Ask permission.* Always ask the wheelchair user if he or she would like assistance before you help. It may be necessary for the person to give you some instructions. An unexpected push could throw the wheelchair user off balance.
2. *Be respectful.* A person's wheelchair is part of his or her body space and should be treated with respect. Don't hang on it unless you have the person's permission.

3. *Speak directly.* Be careful not to exclude the wheelchair user from conversations. Speak directly to the person and if the conversation lasts more than a few minutes, sit down or kneel to get yourself on the same plane as the wheelchair. Also, don't be tempted to pat a person in a wheelchair on the head as it is a degrading gesture.

4. *Give clear directions.* When giving directions to a person in a wheelchair, be sure to include distance, weather conditions, and physical obstacles which may hinder a wheelchair user's travel.

5. *Act natural.* It is okay to use expressions like "running along" when speaking to a person in a wheelchair. It is likely the wheelchair user expresses things the same way.

6. *Wheelchair use doesn't mean confinement.* Be aware that persons who use wheelchairs are not confined to them. When a person transfers to a chair, toilet, car, or other object, do not move the wheelchair out of reaching distance.

7. *Children are O.K..* Don't discourage children from asking questions about wheelchairs and disabilities. Children have a natural curiosity that needs to be satisfied so they do not develop fearful or misleading attitudes. Most wheelchair users are not offended by questions children ask them about their disabilities or wheelchairs.

8. *Some wheelchair users can walk.* Be aware of a wheelchair user's capabilities. Some users can walk with aid, such as braces, walkers, or crutches, and use wheelchairs some of the time to conserve energy and move about more quickly.

9. *Wheelchair users aren't sick.* Don't classify persons who use wheelchairs as sick. Although wheelchairs are often associated with hospitals, they are used for a variety of noncontagious disabilities.

10. *Relationships are important.* Remember that persons in wheelchairs can enjoy fulfilling relationships which may develop into marriage and family. They have physical needs like everyone else.

11. *Wheelchair use provides freedom.* Don't assume that using a wheelchair is in itself a tragedy. It is a means of freedom which allows the user to move about independently. Structural barriers in public places create some inconveniences; however, more and more public places are becoming wheelchair accessible.

(Printed with permission of Schoitz Medical Center, Waterloo, Iowa)

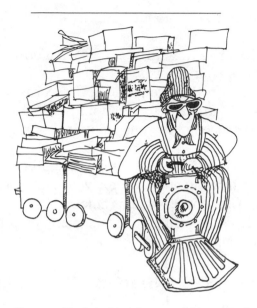

John has discovered he has the right to read his medical records.

YOUR RIGHTS AS A HOSPITAL PATIENT

The American Hospital Association, through the National Society of Patient Representatives of the American Hospital Association, has sent to each state a Patients' and Residents' Bill of Rights with suggestions about how to implement it.

This Bill of Rights has been legislated in only a handful of states, but most hospitals try, at least in some way, to implement it. A copy of the Patients' Bill of Rights is included in the appendix on Finding Help at the end of this book.

Regardless of your age, sex, race, religion, financial situation, and medical condition, you have the right to adequate medical care. This is more than just arranging for you to move if your roommate is too noisy or a chain-smoker. The Patients' Bill of Rights states clearly that you are entitled to the following (see appendix for complete copy):

1. To courteous treatment as a patient.
2. To know who your primary physician is.

3. To get full information about your treatment and other options for treatment.
4. To be allowed privacy with regard to medical treatment as well as confidentiality of your records.
5. To be allowed to review your medical records. (Your care provider, however, has the authority to withhold portions of your record if he or she deems it detrimental to your emotional or physical health.)

Most larger hospitals also have an ombudsman or patient representative. This person has been hired to advocate for your rights as a patient. Don't be shy about discussing your concerns. The role of ombudsman, whether or not that is the official title, is often filled by some member of the hospital staff or a sympathetic social worker.

FINANCIAL ASSISTANCE AND HEALTH INSURANCE

There are many types of financial aid. Basically, they are broken down into four categories.

1. Private medical assistance, such as Blue Cross/Blue Shield or a health maintenance organization (HMO).
2. State assistance, such as welfare, medical assistance, food stamps, and workers' compensation.
3. Federal assistance, such as Medicare, Medicaid, Supplemental Security Income (SSI), Veteran's Administration Assistance, and Social Security.
4. Community assistance, including associations and support groups and information and referral lines.

Private medical assistance: When applying for private insurance, it is imperative to obtain a *major medical policy* which will cover most of your significant medical expenses. In addition to the medical problems you already have, you will need protection for future problems. It is wise to be covered for those large, unforeseen medical expenses.

You may find that some insurance companies will not accept you because of your chronic illness. If you have trouble finding coverage, ask an association or support group in your area for referrals and recommendations.

Regardless of the company you select, always read your policy carefully before signing it. If you have a problem understanding any part of it, get assistance from someone who does. Make sure that the coverage is adequate for your present needs, your anticipated future needs, and the unexpected needs.

The number of health maintenance organizations (HMO's) in the U.S. is growing rapidly. These alternatives to insurance companies cost less than most major medical insurance policies, and their monthly fee is predictable. In contrast to most insurance companies, HMO's generally emphasize preventive health care. This orientation often reduces the need for or duration of hospital visits. There are, however, drawbacks to some health maintenance organizations. You may have fewer physicians to choose from, or your designated clinic or hospital may be inconvenient for you.

In making your decision, you may wish to contact others who have coverage with the insurance company or HMO you are considering. Whatever choice you make, read the small print carefully (about monthly cost, reimbursement method, allowable expenses, approved physicians and clinics, and restrictions). Be sure you feel comfortable with all aspects of the coverage *before* you sign an agreement.

State assistance: State-supported public health care is primarily welfare or medical assistance, but there are many additional programs which your welfare office can give you more information about.

For years, public assistance has been stigmatized by people who have associated it with poverty and lack of education. Don't let that perception stop you from getting the help you need. Public assistance, including food stamps, can make a huge difference.

Food stamps are used as cash for food in a grocery store. They are purchased at a discount so that more food can be purchased. It is unfortunate that so many still don't know that they are eligible for food stamps. Food stamps can make the difference between barely surviving and eating nutritiously. Call your local welfare office for specific information on food stamps.

Workers' compensation: Regardless of what state you live in, if you are injured on your job, call the closest Workers' Compensation Department and ask to file a "first report of injury" report. Tell your employer immediately that you have been injured on the job.

Federal assistance: The federal government offers Medicare, Medicaid, and Veteran's Administration assistance to people who are unable to pay all or part of their medical expenses. The broadest medical coverage is offered under

Medicare. There are several different eligibility options under Medicare, and the amount of coverage varies by the category for which you qualify. If you are over 64, regardless of whether you are eligible for Social Security, you may be eligible for Medicare.

Even if you do not meet the qualifications for Medicare at this time, you may be able to pay a fixed monthly fee and "buy in" to the program. For up-to-date information on Medicare, call your local Medicare office.

If you are unable to afford Medicare, you may be eligible for *Medicaid.* To qualify, you must be 65 or older and on Supplemental Security Income (SSI). See below for more information on SSI. Medicaid is administered by your state, but the federal government requires that some hospital coverage, some X-ray, some laboratory studies, some doctor bills, and some nursing fees may be covered.

For information about Medicaid and eligibility requirements, call your local welfare office.

If you have a chronic illness or medical condition, you may find yourself filing for *Social Security* or *Supplemental Security Income* disability benefits. Very often the specific disease associations have suggestions to help members file a successful application.

You are eligible for Social Security if:

■ You are unable to work because of an illness or injury that is expected to last a year or longer.

■ You are 62 or older and plan to retire.

■ You are within three months of age 65, even if you don't plan to retire.

■ Someone in your family dies.

■ You, your spouse, or your dependent child suffers permanent kidney failure.

To apply for Supplementary Security Income (SSI), you must be over 65 and blind or disabled. SSI defines disabled as having a physical or mental condition which prevents you from doing any substantial gainful work, or is expected to last for at least 12 months, or is expected to result in death.

If your application is denied when you apply for either Social Security or Supplemental Security Income, find out the reasons why so you will have a better chance when you file again or appeal the decision.

Here are the "must read" publications from the Social Security Administration that you should ask for:

A Brief Explanation of Medicare, Publication 05-10035
SSI for Aged, Disabled, and Blind People, Publication 05-10029
Social Security Strengthened, Publication 05-10055

For futher information about Social Security or Supplementary Security Income contact the Social Security office nearest you.

Veteran's Administration Assistance is available to veterans over the age of 64, or any age if you are already on a pension. Call your local Veteran's Administration for more information.

APPENDIX: FINDING HELP

ORGANIZATIONS AND NATIONAL OFFICES, UNITED STATES

Adult Day Care Associations
(consult your local directory or call your local United Way)

Alexander Graham Bell
  Association for the Deaf
3417 Volta Place, N.W.
Washington, DC 20007

American Association of Marriage
  and Family Counselors
225 Yale Avenue
Claremont, CA 91711

American Association on
  Mental Deficiency
1719 Kalorama Rd. N.W.
Washington, DC 20009

American Association for
  Sex Education and Counselors
5010 Wisconsin Avenue N. W.
Suite 304
Washington, DC 20016

American Cancer Society
777 Third Avenue
New York, NY 10017

American Coalition of Citizens
  with Disabilities
1200 15th St., N.W.
Suite 201
Washington, DC 20005

American Diabetes Association
National Service Center
1160 Duke Street
P.O. Box 25757
Alexandria, VA 22314

American Geriatric Society
10 Columbus Circle
Suite 1470
New York, NY 10019

American Heart Association
  National Office
7320 Greenville Avenue
Dallas, TX 75231

American Home Economics
  Association
2010 Massachusetts Avenue, N.W.
Washington, DC 20036

American Lung Association
1740 Broadway
New York, NY 10019

American Lupus Society,
  National Office
23751 Madison Street
Torrance, CA 90505

American Medical Association
535 North Dearborn Street
Chicago, IL 60610

American Occupational Therapy
  Association, Inc.
1383 Piccard Drive
Rockville, MD 20850

American Parkinson Disease
  Association
116 John Street
New York, NY 10038

American Physical Therapy
  Association
1156 15th Street, N.W.
Washington, DC 20005

American Psychiatric Association
1700 18th Street, N.W.
Washington, DC 20009

American Psychological Association
1200 17th Street, N.W.
Washington, DC 20036

American Society of Handicapped
  Physicians (ASHP)
137 Main Street
Grambling, LA 71245
  *(A non-profit organization offering
  assistance to physically handicapped
  people who have chosen a medical
  career. Assistance takes the form of
  support, advocacy, rehabilitation,
  education, employment, and
  communication.)*

American Vocational Association
1510 H Street, N.W.
Washington, DC 20036
  (Career information)

The Amyotrophic Lateral Sclerosis
  Association
185 Madison Avenue, Suite 1001
P.O. Box 2130
New York, NY 10016

Arthritis Foundation-National Office
1314 Spring Street, N.W.
Atlanta, GA 30309

The Association for the Severely
  Handicapped
7010 Roosevelt Way, NE
Seattle, WA 98115

Association of Heart Patients
P.O. Box 54305
Atlanta, GA 30308

Asthma Care Association of America
P.O. Box 568
Spring Valley Road
Ossining, NY 10562

Clearinghouse on the Handicapped
Office of Special Education and
   Rehabilitative Services
Department of Education
Room 3106, Switzer Building
330 C Street, S.W.
Washington, DC 20202

Coronary Club
3659 Green Road
Cleveland, OH 44122

Department of Health, Education
   and Welfare
Social and Rehabilitation Services
Rehabilitation Service
   Administration
Washington, DC 20014

Dysautonomia Foundation, Inc.
370 Lexington Avenue
New York, NY 10017

Epilepsy Foundation of America
4351 Garden Drive
Suite 406
Landover, MD 20785

Family Interest Group-Head
   Trauma
432 Second Street
P.O. 375
Excelsior, MN 55331

Friedreich's Ataxia Group in
   America, Inc.
Box 1116
Oakland, CA 94611

Gerontological Society
Clinical Medicine Section
1 Dupont Circle
Washington, DC 20036

Gullian-Barré Syndrome
   Support Group
P.O. 262
Wynnewood, PA 19096

Hospice Organizations
   *(consult your local directory or call
   your local United Way)*

HOW
Handicapped Organized Women
P.O. Box 35481
Charlotte, NC 28235
   *(A newly-formed organization acting
   as a support group and outreach
   organization for handicapped
   women. State chapters now forming.)*

Library of Congress
Division for the Blind and Physically
   Handicapped
Washington, DC 20542

The Lupus Foundation of America,
   Inc., National Office
P.O. Box 12897
St. Louis, MO 63141

Muscular Dystrophy Association,
   National Office
810 Seventh Avenue
New York, NY 10019

Myasthenia Gravis Foundation, Inc.
7-11 South Broadway, Suite 304
White Plains, NY 10601

National Association for the Deaf
814 Thayer Avenue
Silver Springs, MD 20907

National Association of
   Social Workers
1425 H Street, N.W., Suite 600
Washington, DC 20005

National Association of the
   Physically Handicapped
2810 Terrace Road S.E.
Washington, DC 20020

National Ataxia Foundation
600 Twelve Oaks Center
15500 Wayzata Boulevard
Wayzata, MN 55391

National Cancer Institute
9000 Rockville Pike
Bethesda, MD 20892
For info: call 1-800-4-Cancer
For pamphlets: 1-800-638-6694

National Center for a Barrier Free
   Environment
1140 Connecticut Avenue, N.W.
Suite 1006
Washington, DC 20036

National Heart and Lung Institute
Bethesda, MD 20014

National Institute of Mental Health
5600 Fishers Lane
Rockville, MD 20852

National Lupus Erythematosus
   Foundation
5430 Van Nuys Boulevard, Suite 206
Van Nuys, CA 91401

National Multiple Sclerosis Society,
   National Office
208 East 42nd Street
New York, NY 10017

National Myoclonus Foundation
845 Third Avenue
New York, NY 10022

National Organization for
   Rare Disorders, Inc.
P.O. Box 8923
New Fairfield, Conn. 06812

National Psoriasis Foundation Inc.
6415 S.W. Canyon Court, Suite 200
Portland, OR 97221

National Rehabilitation Association
633 South Washington Street
Alexandria, VA 22314

National Rehabilitation
   Information Center
4407 Eighth Street, NE
The Catholic University of America
Washington, DC 20017

National Self-Help Clearinghouse
Graduate School & University Center
   of the City University of New
   York
33 West 42nd Street, Room 1227
New York, NY 10036

Parkinson's Educational Program
(PEP*USA)
1800 Park Newport, #302
Newport Beach, CA 92660
*(A wide variety of products and
information resources; write for
complete catalog and newsletter.)*

President's Commission on Employment of the Handicapped
1111 20th St., N. W., Suite 636
Washington, DC 20036

Sex Information and Education
Council of the U. S. (SIECUS)
80 Fifth Avenue, Suite 801-2
New York, NY 10011

Sex Information and Education
Council of the U. S. (SIECUS)
New York University Resource
Center and Library
51 West 4th Street
New York, NY 10003
*(This is an excellent resource for lay
people and professionals. Request the
complete list of available topics.)*

Sister Kenny Institute
800 E. 28th St. at Chicago Ave.
Minneapolis, MN 55407

Tourette Syndrome Association
41-02 Bell Boulevard
Bayside, NY 11361

United Scleroderma Foundation
P.O. Box 724
Watsonville, CA 95076

Vocational Guidance and
Rehabilitation Services
2289 East 55th Street
Cleveland, OH 44103

ORGANIZATIONS AND NATIONAL OFFICES, CANADA

ALS Society of Canada
(Amyotrophic Lateral Sclerosis)
250 Rogers Road
Toronto, Ontario M6E 1R1
Canada

Arthritis Society (Canada)
Suite 420
920 Younge Street
Toronto, Ontario, M4W 3J7
Canada

Autism Society of Canada
P.O. Box 472
Station A
Scarborough, Ontario M1K 5C3
Canada

Canadian National Institute
  for the Blind
1931 Bayview Avenue
Toronto, Ontario M4G 4C8
Canada

Canadian Association for the Deaf
2395 Bayview Avenue
Willowdale, Ontario M2L 1A2

Canadian Association for Narcolepsy
P.O. Box 193
Station S
Toronto, Ontario M5M 4L7
Canada

Canadian Cancer Society
130 Bloor Street West, Suite 1001
Toronto, Ontario M5S 2V7
Canada

Canadian Cystic Fibrosis Foundation
586 Eglinton Avenue East
Suite 204
Toronto, Ontario M5S 1N5
Canada

Canadian Diabetes Association
78 Bond Street
Toronto, Ontario M5B 2J8
Canada

Canadian Foundation for
  Ileitis and Colitis
294 Spadina Avenue
Toronto, Ontario M5T 2E7
Canada

Canadian Heart and Stroke
  Foundation
1 Nicholas Street, Suite 1200
Ottawa, Ontario K1N 7B7
Canada

Canadian Lung Association
75 Albert Street
Suite 908
Ottawa, Ontario K1P 5E7
Canada

C.M.T. International
  (Charcot-Marie-Tooth Syndrome)
34-B Bayview Drive
St. Catharines, Ontario L2N 4Y6
Canada

Epilepsy Ontario
2160 Yonge Street, First Floor
Toronto, Ontario M4S 2A9
Canada

Lupus Foundation of Ontario
  Corporation
P.O. Box 687
289 Ridge Road North
Ridgeway, Ontario L0S 1N0
Canada

Multiple Sclerosis Society of Canada
130 Bloor Street West, Suite 700
Toronto, Ontario M5S 1S5
Canada

Muscular Dystrophy
   Association of Canada
357 Bay Street, Tenth Floor
Toronto, Ontario M5H 2T7
Canada

Ontario March of Dimes
   (Crippling Illnesses)
60 Overlea Boulevard
Toronto, Ontario M4H 1B6
Canada

Parkinson Foundation of Canada
232 55 Bloor Street West
Toronto, Ontario M4W 1A6
Canada

PRODUCTS AND SERVICES

Abbey Medical Catalog Sales
13782 Crenshaw Blvd.
Gardena, CA 90249
800-262-1294 (toll free in California)
800-421-5126 (toll free in other
   states)

R. G. Abernathy, Inc.
Route 1, Box 1
Creston, NC 28615
800-334-0128 (Custom shoes)

ABLE DATA
National Rehabilitation
   Information Center
4407 Eighth Street, N.E.
Washington, DC 20017
(202) 635-6090
(202) 635-5884 (TTP)
   *(This is a computerized national data
   base for rehabilitation products)*

Accent on Living Magazine
Gillum Road and High Drive
P.O. Box 700
Bloomington, IL 61702
   *(Supplier to the disabled and
   chronically ill; write for catalog)*

Access Travel: A Guide to
   Accessibility
   of Airport Terminals
U.S. General Services
   Administration
Washington, DC 20405

Accurate Medical Service
8004 West Chester Pike
Upper Darby, PA 19082

Air Travel for the Handicapped
TWA
605 Third Avenue
New York, NY 10016

Air Travelers Fly Rights
Office of Consumer Affairs
Civil Aeronautics Board
Washington, DC 20428

(AIS) Appliance Information Service
Whirlpool Corporation
Administrative Center
Benton Harbor, MI 49022
   *(Ask for "Designs for Independent
   Living" and other booklets)*

Alda Industries, Inc.
214 Harvard Avenue
Boston, MA 02134
   *(E-Z up chair to help people who
   have difficulty with sitting or getting
   out of a chair)*

Amigo Sales, Inc.
6693 Dixie Highway
Bridgeport, MI 48603

American Automobile Association
1712 G. Street N. W.
Washington, DC 20015
   *(Free list of automobile hand-control
   manufacturers)*

American Podiatry Association
20 Chevy Chase Circle, N.W.
Washington, DC 20015

Arthritis Centers (Multipurpose)
   *(Network of 21 centers throughout
   the U.S. Call your State Arthritis
   Foundation to see if one is located
   near your home.)*

Arthritis Information Clearinghouse
P.O. Box 9782
Arlington, VA 22209
   *(NOT for the general public, but
   they will provide addresses and
   sources of where to purchase or write
   for articles and books. Write for the
   "Patient Education Resource on the
   Rheumatic Diseases" catalog.)*

Battle Creek Equipment
307 West Jackson Street
Battle Creek, MI 49017-2385
800-253-0854
   *(Request catalog of equipment from
   exercise bikes to an automatic moist
   heat pack)*

Bird and Cronin, Inc.
Home Health Care Centers
508 Jackson Street
St. Paul, MN 55101
   *(Write for "Home Health Care"
   catalog)*

Birkenstock Shoes
46 Galli Drive
Vorato, CA 94947
   (Write for current shoe catalog)

A.R. Bolz
3939 Cloverhill Road
Baltimore, MD 21218
   *(Sleeves to filter ultraviolet light from
   fluorescent lights)*

Brookstone Company
127 Vose Farm Road
Peterborough, NH 03458
   *(Write for catalog on hard-
   to-find tools and other fine
   things)*

Bruce Medical Supply
411 Waverly Oaks Road
Waltham, MA 02154
   *(Mail order medical and daily living
   supplies)*

Care Chair Systems, Inc.
5602 Elmwood Avenue
Indianapolis, IN 46203

Care Company Equipment, Inc.
66 Commerce Street
Thornwood, NY

Chronic Pain Letter
Box 1303
Old Chelsea Station
New York, NY 10011
   *(Newsletter reports on therapies,
   medications, aids, studies, clinics,
   and more)*

Cleo Living Aids
3957 Mayfield Road
Cleveland, OH 44121
   *(Write for catalog on daily living
   aids including bath and shower
   devices)*

C.M.T. Newsletter
(Charcot-Marie-Tooth syndrome)
34 B Bayview Drive
St. Catherines, Ontario
Canada L2N 4Y6
   (A quarterly for those with CMT)

Comfortably Yours
52 West Hunter Avenue
Maywood, NJ 07607
   *(Write for catalog on aids for easier
   living)*

Consumer Product Information
   Service
Public Documents Distribution
   Center
Pueblo, CO 81009

Joan Cook
3200 S. E. 14th Avenue
Ft. Lauderdale, FL 33316
   (Gadgets and aids)

Cosco Home Products
2525 State Street
Columbus, IN 47201

Diabetes Center, Inc.
13911 Ridgedale Drive, Suite 250
Minneapolis, MN 55343
   *(Write for product and service
   catalog)*

Disability and Chronic Disease
   Quarterly (newsletter)
Irving K. Zola
Brandeis University
Department of Sociology
Waltham, MA 02254

Earl's Stairway Lift Corporation
2513 Center Street
Highway 218 North
Cedar Falls, IA 50613

Elder Ensembles
7400 Metro Blvd., Suite 410
Edina, MN 55435
 (Adapted clothing and shoe service, catalog, convenience items)

Enrichments: Helping Hands for
 Special Needs
P.O. Box 579
145 Tower Drive
Hinsdale, IL 60921

Everest and Jennings
3233 E. Mission Oaks Blvd.
Camarillo, CA 93010
 (Wheelchairs, home and hospital medical supplies)

Fashion-Able, Inc.
Rock Hill, NJ 08553
 (Write for adaptive clothing catalog, mail order clothes for women)

Foley Manufacturing Company
Housewares Division
3300 N. E. 5th Street
Minneapolis, MN 55418

Gandy Company
528 Gandrud Road
Owatonna, MD 55060
 (Special four-wheel bike for extra stability)

Grass Roots Promotions
Dept. W
322 West Roosevelt Street
Freeport, IL 61032
 ("Rest-Stop" seat to put on walker)

Hammacher Schlemmer
145 East 57th Street
New York, NY 10022
 (Catalog for gadgets and aids for living)

Handi-Ramp, Inc.
1414 Armour Boulevard
Mundelein, IL 60060

Hapad, Inc.
P.O. Box 6
5301 Enterprise Boulevard
Bethel Park, PA 15102
 (Felt-pads to help relieve pressure points on painful feet)

Headstrom Company
P.O. Box 156
Glendale, AZ 85311
 (Tricycle for added stability while exercising)

Helping Hand Service for the
 Handicapped
Greyhound Lines
Greyhound Towers
Phoenix, AZ 85077

HUSA Folding Crutch Co., Inc.
6 Dravus Street
Seattle, WA 98109
 (Aluminum folding crutches)

Kagle Surgical Supply Co.
4422 Bronx Blvd.
Bronx, NY 10470

Miles Kimball
Kimball Building
41 West 8th Avenue
Oshkosh, WI 54901
   *(Catalog of gadgets and practical
   devices)*

Maddak, Inc.
Pequannock, NJ 07440
   *(Write for catalog of home health
   care equipment, "Special products
   for people with special needs")*

Mainstream
Magazine of the ABLE-DISABLED
P.O. Box 2781
Escondido, CA 92025

Mainstream, Inc.
1200 15th Street, N.W., Suite 403
Washington, DC 20005
202-833-1160
   *(A non-profit organization seeking to
   provide better employment for the
   disabled)*

Medic Alert Foundation
   International
P.O. Box 1009
Turlock, CA 95380
209-634-4917 (call collect)
   *(A confidential, 24-hour medical
   information service providing
   emergency information related*

*to members' medical conditions; free
medical information bracelet or
necklace provided with membership
fee)*

Jerry Miller I.D. Shoes
Marble Street
Whitman, MA 02382
   (Custom-molded shoes)

Montgomery Ward
Albany, NY 12201
   *(Write for home health care catalog
   or call local store)*

National Odd Shoe Exchange
Rural Route 4
Indianola, IA 50125

Nelson Medical Products
5690 Sarah Avenue
Sarasota, FL 33581

Northern Wire Products, Inc.
P.O. Box 70 West Div. Street
St. Cloud, MN 56302
   *("Backjack" seat for back support;
   multiple uses, portable)*

Office for Handicapped Individuals
Department of Health, Education
   and Welfare
200 Independence Ave. S.W.
Washington, DC 20201

Office of Consumer Affairs
Civil Aeronautics Board
Washington, DC 20428
   (Ask for "Air Traveler's Fly
   Rights")

Patient to Patient:
A Health Education Newsletter
P.O. Box 16294
St. Paul, MN 55116
   (A subscription newsletter to enhance
   awareness of adaptive living aids)

Physical Aids Marketing Company
144 South Orange Avenue
El Cajon, CA 92020

Plasti-Dip International
1458 West Country Road C.
St. Paul, MN 55113
   (Product to dip and cover handles
   with rubber-like substance for easier
   gripping)

Quadra Wheelchairs, Inc.
3117 Via Colinas
Westlake Village, CA 91362
   (Wheelchairs with equipment
   including adjustable armrests)

Reader Enterprises, Inc.
193 Robinson Street
Binghamton, NY 13904
   ("No Hands" Reading Stand)

Rehabilitation Equipment and
   Supply
1823 West Moss Avenue
Peoria, IL 61606

Rehabilitation International, USA
1123 Broadway, Suite 704, Box PR
New York, NY 10010
   (Write for "International Directory
   of Access Guide" for disabled
   travelers; send stamped business
   envelope)

Roloke Company
P.O. Box 24DD3
Los Angeles, CA 90024
   (Healthcare products including Wal-
   Pil-O and chair leg extenders to ease
   the strain of sitting and rising)

Rubbermaid, Inc.
1147 Akron Road
Wooster, OH 44691
   (Kitchen and other household
   equipment)

Sabel Shoe Company
Benson-East Room 107
Jenkintown, PA 19046
   (Extra-depth thermal-molded shoe)

Fred Sammons, Inc.
Box 32
Brookfield, IL 60513
   (Write for catalogs on daily living
   aids)

Sci-Tech
501 Richardson Drive
Lancaster, PA 17603
800-233-0291
   (A lift seat chair that looks just like a
   recliner)

Sears Roebuck and Company
4640 Roosevelt Blvd.
Philadelphia, PA 19321
  (Write the headquarters or call the catalog desk of your local store)

Southeastern Mobility
  Company, Inc.
8236 Middlebrook Pike
Knoxville, TN 37919

Spencer Gifts
Atlantic City, NJ 08411
  (Gadgets and aids for living)

Sunset House
12800 Culver Blvd.
Los Angeles, CA 90066
  (A gadget catalog for easier living plus fun items)

Swing-A-Way
  Manufacturing Company
4100 Beck Avenue
St. Louis, MO 63116
  (small kitchen devices)

Timely Products Corporation
860 Honeyspot Road
Stratford, CN 06497

Unique Products
340 Popular Street
Hanover, PA 17331

U.S. General Services
  Administration
Washington, DC 20405
  (Write for "Access Travel: A Guide to Accessibility of Airport Terminals")

U.S. Government Printing Office
Washington, DC 20402
  (Ask for list of topics related to your illness, including "Clothing Tips for the Woman with Arthritis")

Velcro Corporation
681 Fifth Avenue
New York, NY 10022
  (Write for a catalog on the uses of velcro)

Ways and Means
28001 Citrin Drive
Romulus, MI 48174
  (Write for catalog for access to over 1000 adaptive aids and general use products for daily living)

Winco Products
Winfield Company, Inc.
3062 46th Avenue, North
St. Petersburg, FL 33714
  (Self-help equipment)

Zim Manufacturing Company
2850 West Fulton Street
Chicago, IL 60612
  (Write for a catalog including the Zim jar opener)

PATIENTS' AND RESIDENTS' BILL OF RIGHTS (MINNESOTA)

Legislative Intent: It is the intent of the legislature and the purpose of this section to promote the interests and well-being of the patients and residents of health care facilities. No health care facility may require a patient or resident to waive these rights as a condition of admission to the facility. Any guardian or conservator of a patient or resident or, in the absence of a guardian or conservator, an interested person, may seek enforcement of these rights on behalf of a patient or resident. An interested person may also seek enforcement of these rights on behalf of a patient or resident who has a guardian or conservator through administrative agencies or in probate court or county court having jurisdiction over guardianships and conservatorships. Pending the outcome of an enforcement proceeding the health care facility may, in good faith, comply with the instructions of a guardian or conservator. It is the intent of this section that every patient's civil and religious liberties, including the right to independent personal decisions and knowledge of available choices, shall not be infringed and that the facility shall encourage and assist in the fullest possible exercise of these rights.

Definitions: For the purposes of this section, "patient" means a person who is admitted to an acute care inpatient facility for a continuous period longer than 24 hours, for the purpose of diagnosis or treatment bearing on the physical or mental health of that person. "Resident" means a person who is admitted to a non-acute care facility including extended care facilities, nursing homes, and board and care homes for care required because of prolonged mental or physical illness or disability, recovery from injury or disease, or advancing age.

Public Policy Declaration: It is declared to be the public policy of this state that the interests of each patient and resident be protected by a declaration of a patients' bill of rights which shall include but not be limited to the rights specified in this section.

1. *Information About Rights:* Patients and residents shall, at admission, be told that there are legal rights for their protection during their stay at the facility and that these are described in an accompanying written statement of the applicable rights and responsibilities set forth in this section. Reasonable arrangements shall be made for those with communication impairments and those who speak a language other than

English. Current facility policies, inspection findings of state and local health authorities, and further explanation of the written statement of rights shall be available to patients, residents, their guardians or their chosen representatives upon reasonable request to the administrator or other designated staff person.

2. *Courteous Treatment:* Patients and residents have the right to be treated with courtesy and respect for their individuality by employees of or persons providing service in a health care facility.

3. *Appropriate Health Care:* Patients and residents shall have the right to appropriate medical and personal care based on individual needs. Appropriate care for residents means care designed to enable residents to achieve their highest level of physical and mental functioning. This right is limited where the service is not reimbursable by public or private resources.

4. *Physician's Identity:* Patients and residents shall have or be given, in writing, the name, business address, telephone number, and specialty, if any, of the physician responsible for coordination of their care. In cases where it is medically inadvisable, as documented by the attending physician in a patient's or resident's care record, the information shall be given to the patient's or resident's guardian or other person designated by the patient or resident as his or her representative.

5. *Relationship With Other Health Services:* Patients and residents who receive services from an outside provider are entitled, upon request, to be told the identity of the provider. Residents shall be informed, in writing, of any health care services which are provided to those residents by individuals, corporations, or organizations other than their facility. Information shall include the name of the outside provider, the address, and a description of the service which may be rendered. In cases where it is medically inadvisable as documented by the attending physician in a patient's or resident's care record, the information shall be given to the patient's or resident's guardian or other person designated by the patient or resident as his or her representative.

6. *Information About Treatment:* Patients and residents shall be given by their physicians complete and current information concerning their diagnosis, treatment, alternatives, risks, and prognosis as required by the physician's legal duty to disclose. This information shall be in terms and language the patients or residents can reasonably be expected to understand. Patients and residents may be accompanied by a family member or other chosen representative. This information shall include the likely medical or major psychological results of the treatment and its alternatives. In cases where it is medically inadvisable, as documented by the attending physician in a patient's or resident's medical record, the information shall be given to the patient's or resident's guardian or other person designated by the patient or resident as his or her representative. Individuals have the right to refuse this information.

Every patient or resident suffering from any form of breast cancer shall be fully informed, prior to or at the time of admission and during her stay, of all alternative effective methods of treatment of which the treating physician is knowledgeable, including surgical, radiological, or chemotherapeutic treatments or combinations of treatments and the risks associated with each of those methods.

7. *Participation in Planning Treatment:* Patients and residents shall have the right to participate in the planning of their health care. This right includes the opportunity to discuss treatment and alternatives with individual caregivers, the opportunity to request and participate in formal care conferences, and the right to include a family member or other chosen representative. In the event that the patient or resident cannot be present, a family member or other representative chosen by the patient or resident may be included in such conferences.

8. *Continuity of Care.* Patients and residents shall have the right to be cared for with reasonable regularity and continuity of staff assignment as far as facility policy allows.

9. *Right to Refuse Care:* Competent patients and residents shall have the right to refuse treatment based on the information required in Right No. 6. Residents who refuse treatment, medication, or dietary

restrictions shall be informed of the likely medical or major psychological results of the refusal, with documentation in the individual medical record. In cases where a patient or resident is incapable of understanding the circumstances but has not been adjudicated incompetent, or when legal requirements limit the right to refuse treatment, the conditions and circumstances shall be fully documented by the attending physician in the patient's or resident's medical record.

10. *Experimental Research:* Written, informed consent must be obtained prior to a patient's or resident's participation in experimental research. Patients and residents have the right to refuse participation. Both consent and refusal shall be documented in the individual care record.

11. *Freedom from Abuse:* Patients and residents shall be free from mental and physical abuse as defined in the Vulnerable Adults Protection Act. "Abuse" means any act which constitutes assault, sexual exploitation, or criminal sexual conduct as described in section 626.557, subdivision 2d, or the intentional and nontherapeutic infliction of physical pain or injury, or any persistent course of conduct intended to produce mental or emotional distress. Every patient and resident shall also be free from nontherapeutic chemical and physical restraints, except in fully documented emergencies, or as authorized in writing after examination by a patient's or resident's physician for a specified and limited period of time, and only when necessary to protect the patient or resident from self-injury or injury to others.

12. *Treatment Privacy:* Patients and residents shall have the right to respectfulness and privacy as it relates to their medical and personal care program. Case discussion, consultation, examination, and treatment are confidential and shall be conducted discreetly. Privacy shall be respected during toileting, bathing, and other activities of personal hygiene, except as needed for patient or resident safety or assistance.

13. *Confidentiality of Records:* Patients and residents shall be assured confidential treatment of their personal and medical records, and may approve or refuse their release to any individual outside the facility. Residents shall be notified when personal records are requested by any

individual outside the facility and may select someone to accompany them when the records or information are the subject of a personal interview. Copies of records and written information from the records shall be made available in accordance with this subdivision and section 144.335. This right does not apply to complaint investigations and inspections by the department of health, where required by third party payment contracts, or where otherwise provided by law.

14. *Disclosure of Services Available:* Patients and residents shall be informed, prior to or at the time of admission and during their stay, of services which are included in the facility's basic per diem or daily room rate and that other services are available at additional charges. Facilities shall make every effort to assist patients and residents in obtaining information regarding whether the medicare or medical assistance program will pay for any or all of the aforementioned services.

15. *Responsive Service:* Patients and residents shall have the right to a prompt and reasonable response to their questions and requests.

16. *Personal Privacy:* Patients and residents shall have the right to every consideration of their privacy, individuality, and cultural identity as related to their social, religious, and psychological well-being. Facility staff shall respect the privacy of a resident's room by knocking on the door and seeking consent before entering, except in an emergency or where clearly inadvisable.

17. *Grievances:* Patients and residents shall be encouraged and assisted throughout their stay in a facility, to understand and exercise their rights as patients, residents, and citizens. Patients and residents may voice grievances and recommend changes in policies and services to facility staff and others of their choice, free from restraint, interference, coercion, discrimination, or reprisal, including threat of discharge. Notice of the facility's grievance procedure, as well as addresses and telephone numbers for the office of health facility complaints and the area nursing home ombudsman pursuant to the Older Americans Act, section 307(a)(12) shall be posted in a conspicuous place.

18. *Communication Privacy:* Patients and residents may associate and communicate privately with persons of their choice and enter and, except as provided by the Minnesota Commitment Act, leave the facility as they choose. Patients and residents shall have access, at their expense, to writing instruments, stationery, and postage. Personal mail shall be sent without interference and received unopened unless medically or programmatically contraindicated and documented by the physician in the medical record. There shall be access to a telephone where patients and residents can make and receive calls as well as speak privately. Facilities which are unable to provide a private area shall make reasonable arrangements to accommodate the privacy of patients' or residents' calls. This right is limited where medically inadvisable, as documented by the attending physician in a patient's or resident's care record. Where programmatically limited by a facility abuse prevention plan pursuant to the Vulnerable Adults Protection Act, section 626.557, subdivision 14, clause 2, this right shall also be limited accordingly.

19. *Personal Property:* Patients and residents may retain and use their personal clothing and possessions as space permits, unless to do so would infringe upon rights of other patients or residents, and unless medically or programmatically contraindicated for documented medical, safety, or programmatic reasons. The facility must either maintain a central locked depository or provide individual locked storage areas in which residents may store their valuables for safekeeping. The facility may, but is not required to, provide compensation for or replacement of lost or stolen items.

20. *Services for the Facility:* Patients and residents shall not perform labor or services for the facility unless those activities are included for the therapeutic purposes and appropriately goal related in their individual medical record.

21. *Choice of Supplier:* A resident may purchase or rent goods or services not included in the per diem rate from a supplier of his or her choice unless otherwise provided by law. The supplier shall ensure that these purchases are sufficient to meet the medical or treatment needs of the resident.

22. *Financial Affairs:* Competent residents may manage their personal financial affairs, or shall be given at least a quarterly accounting of financial transactions on their behalf if they delegate this responsibility in accordance with the laws of Minnesota to the facility for any period of time.

23. *Right to Associate:* Residents may meet with visitors and participate in activities of commercial, religious, political, as defined in section 203B.11 and community groups without interference at their discretion if the activities do not infringe on the right to privacy of other residents or are not programmatically contraindicated. This includes the right to join with other individuals within and outside the facility to work for improvements in long-term care.

24. *Advisory Councils:* Residents and their families shall have the right to organize, maintain, and participate in resident advisory and family councils. Each facility shall provide assistance and space for meetings. Council meetings shall be afforded privacy, with staff or visitors attending only upon the council's invitation. A staff person shall be designated the responsibility of providing this assistance and responding to written requests which result from council meetings. Resident and family councils shall be encouraged to make recommendations regarding facility policies.

25. *Married Residents:* Residents, if married, shall be assured privacy for visits by their spouses and, if both spouse are residents of the facility, they shall be permitted to share a room, unless medically contraindicated and documented by their physicians in the medical records.

26. *Transfers and Discharges:* Residents shall not be arbitrarily transferred or discharged. Residents must be notified, in writing, of the proposed discharge or transfer and its justification no later than 30 days before discharge from the facility and seven days before transfer to another room within the facility. This notice shall include the resident's right to contest the proposed action, with the address and telephone number of the area nursing home ombudsman pursuant to the Older Americans Act, section 307(a)(12). The resident, informed

of this right, may choose to relocate before the notice period ends. The notice period may be shortened in situations outside the facility's control, such as a determination by utilization review, the accommodation of newly-admitted residents, a change in the resident's own or another resident's welfare, or nonpayment for stay unless prohibited by the public program or programs paying for the resident's care, as documented in the medical record. Facilities shall make a reasonable effort to accommodate new residents without disrupting room assignments.

Inquiries or complaints regarding medical treatment or the Patients and Residents Bill of Rights for Minnesota may be directed to your state board of medical examiners or office of health facility complaints.

GLOSSARY

Abduction: Movement of the extremities away from the midline of the body.

Adaptive Device: A common article (e.g. a fork) made more suitable for a specific individual or group of individuals.

Adduction: Movement of the extremities toward the midline of the body.

Advocate: To support or plead in favor of; a person who advocates.

Agrypniaphobia: Fear of insomnia.

Alopecia: Hair loss.

Anemia: Deficiency of red blood cells which may be caused by disease or loss of blood.

Anterior: Located at the front of the body.

Anti-inflammatory: An agent that counteracts the inflammatory process.

Ankylosing Spondylitis: A form of arthritis which affects the spine and can cause fixation of the spine.

Aphasia: A total or partial loss of the power to use or understand words.

Arthralgia: Joint pain.

Avascular Necrosis: A condition in which vessels that supply blood to bone become inflamed and bones begin to degenerate causing considerable pain.

Auto-Immune Disorder: A condition in which the body literally attacks itself by making antibodies against its own cells.

Biofeedback: Literally "self-feedback," a method of learning to control bodily functions with audible or visual electrical feedback.

Bradykinesia: Slowness of movement or sluggish physical response.

Butterfly Rash: The classic rash of lupus which covers the bridge of the nose and the cheeks in a butterfly pattern.

Chiropractic: A method of treatment that teaches that all maladies are caused by nerve pressure in the spine and can be helped by spinal adjustment.

Chiropractor: A person who practices chiropractic.

Chronic: Long-standing, usually for life.

Collagen Disease: A disease of the connective tissue in the body.

Connective Tissue: The tissue that binds the body together, found in abundance in every area of the body.

Consultant: A specialist, in this context usually a physician to whom a patient goes for a second opinion on a medical condition.

Coping Mechanism: Emotion or attitude which helps a person deal with stress.

Cortisone: A hormone produced by the cortex of the adrenal glands which can also be produced synthetically.

Covert: Hidden, not obvious.

Crohn's Disease: An inflammatory disease involving any part of the gastrointestinal tract from mouth to anus, but most common in terminal ileum. Has a high rate of reoccurrence.

Cunnilingus: Using the mouth and tongue to stimulate the female's sexual organs.

Depression: A psychiatric syndrome which may be characterized by mood change, sleep problems, weight change, guilt feelings, or feelings of helplessness.

Dermatomyositis: A disease characterized by chronic inflammation of the skin and muscles.

Diabetes: A term referring to disorders characterized by excessive urine secretion. There are two major types: Type I and Type II.

Dildo: A penis-shaped device.

Disability: Loss of ability to carry out specific functions.

Discoid Lupus: A type of lupus in which disc-shaped lesions form over the skin. Butterfly rash may be present, and skin becomes red, crusted, and patchy.

Dyskinesia: The impairment in the power of voluntary movement.

Dyspareunia: Painful or difficult intercourse.

Dysphasia: The impairment of speech or of the ability to understand language.

Endogenous: Originating from inside the body.

Endometritis: Chronic inflammation of the endometrium, which is the inner mucous membrane of the uterus.

Endorphin: A pain control substance, similar to morphine, produced by the human body.

Epicritic: Very sudden reaction to pain, such as would happen with a stubbed toe.

Etiology: The study of factors that cause disease or the origin of disease.

Euphoria: An abnormal or exaggerated sense of well-being.

Exacerbation: An active or acute episode of a disease or condition; a flare.

Exogenous: Originating from outside the body.

Fellatio: Using the mouth and tongue to manipulate or stimulate the penis.

Fibromyalgia: A rheumatoid condition that causes pain and stiffness in the tissues around the joints.

Fibrositis: Pain, stiffness of the deep tissues (not involving the joints).

Friedrich's Ataxia: A slowly progressing disorder of the muscles and the nervous system which cause inability to coordinate movement of the voluntary muscles.

Gel Phenomenon: Morning stiffness, or stiffness after being in one position for a long while.

Gout: A disease in which an excess of uric acid is in the blood, which causes painful inflammation of a joint and which may manifest as chronic arthritis.

Group Therapy: Therapy through which people can begin to be aware of their own problems through group interaction with other people in similar situations, and where other people can often find solutions to problems with the help of others.

Heberdon's Node: Bony knobs which can form around the last joint of the fingers.

Hypnosis: An induced sleep-like state. A person can be hypnotized or learn self-hypnosis.

Ill: Not well, sick.

Imaging: Reproduction of part of a person, such as the brain. Often used as a diagnostic study.

Immunology: Specialization in the study of infectious diseases and the development of immunity.

Insomnia: Trouble getting to sleep or staying asleep.

Internist: A physician who specializes in adult internal diseases.

Kinesics: The science of body language.

Multiple Sclerosis: A chronic, sometimes disabling disease of the central nervous system which can interfere with the brain's ability to control functions such as walking, talking, and seeing.

Muscular Dystrophy: A group of related diseases characterized by weakness and progressive wasting of the skeletal muscles.

Myalgia: Muscle pain.

Myasthenia Gravis: A chronic muscle disease characterized by weakness and extreme fatigue of the voluntary muscles.

Myositis: Fibrositis within the muscles.

Myotonia: A condition in which voluntary muscles are slow to relax after contracting, and can stiffen and be difficult to move.

Myotonic Dystrophy: Progressive wasting of the voluntary muscles.

Nephrologist: A physician who has specialized in conditions involving the kidneys.

Neuritis: Inflammation of the nerves outside of the central nervous system.

Neurologist: A physician who has specialized in conditions involving the nervous system.

Neuropathy: Any disease of the nerves.

Nurse: A person who is specially prepared in the scientific basis of nursing, and who meets certain prescribed standards of education and clinical competence.

Nurturing: The act of nourishing or nursing.

Nutritionist: A person who has specialized in how food nourishes.

Occupational Therapy: Therapy which includes activities needed for daily living or work.

Orthosis: A device, usually a brace or support, custom-built for the purpose of holding straight or straightening a deformed limb or part of the body.

Orthotist: One who makes an orthosis.

Osteoarthritis: Another form of arthritis, often occurring in older people when cartilage around the bone frays or wears and bone rubs against bone.

Overt: Open, obvious.

Parkinson's Disease: A disorder of body movement causing rigidity, tremor and difficulty or slowness of movement.

Pericarditis: Inflammation of the outer membrane surrounding the heart.

Pharmacist: Specialist in compounding drugs (filling medical prescriptions).

Photosensitivity: Hypersensitivity of the skin to sunlight.

Pleurisy: Infection of the lining of the lungs.

Pleuritis: Inflammation of the lining of the lungs.

Physical Therapist: Person trained to help the patient regain strength, movement, coordination, range of motion, and endurance, and possibly to help delay some deformities.

Polymalgia Rheumatica: Rheumatic pain in many muscles.

Polymyositis: Degenerative changes which occur in voluntary muscles, sometimes accompanied by inflammation.

Posterior: Located at the back of the body.

Primary Physician: The physician who coordinates all of a patient's medical care.

Prodrome: Symptoms indicating the approach of a disease.

Prognosis: A prediction of the outcome of a disease.

Proteinuria: Protein in the urine.

Protopathic: Pain which occurs more slowly, such as any pain which has been of long duration.

Psoriatic Arthritis: Arthritis which can accompany psoriasis.

Psychoanalyst: A psychiatrist who specializes is psychoanalysis and who works with patients and their past emotional experiences to help discover why a past pathologic mental state has been produced.

Psychiatrist: A physician who is trained in psychiatry and who treats mental and neurotic disorders and the changes that occur with them.

Psychologist: A person who has specialized in the mental processes and their effect on behavior. The psychologist can help the patient or the patient's family cope with problems, disease, sudden illness, and accidents.

Raynaud's Phenomenon: Coldness of fingers due to poor circulation in the small arteries, which can cause fingers to turn blue or to blanch.

Relaxation Therapy: Therapy, often self-conducted, in which total body relaxation is accomplished according to a specific plan.

Remission: When the symptoms of a disease spontaneously disappear, not as a result of any medicine being used to treat the disease.

Rheumatic: Pertaining to rheumatism, any disorder of the back or extremities.

Rheumatoid Arthritis: Chronic inflammatory disease of the joints and joint membranes which can cause permanent damage to the joint.

Rheumatologist: An internist who has specialized in diseases of the joints.

Rigidity: Stiffness.

Scleroderma: A connective tissue disease in which the skin and/or the internal organs become hard and leathery.

Secondary Physician: A physician who a patient sees, who is separate from his primary physician (e.g. cardiologist, rheumatologist).

Sedimentation Rate: A blood test to determine erythrocyte sedimentation rate, or how red cells sink within the blood over a certain period of time; patients with active inflammatory disease or infections often have elevated sedimentation rates.

Sign: An objective medical finding, usually by examination or by diagnostic testing.

Sjogren's Syndrome: A condition characterized by dryness of the eyes, mouth, throat, and other mucous membranes.

Social Service Worker: A specialist in social work who works with the patient or his family with their problems; in this context, often related to illness, medical care, financial problems, or other family crises.

Specialist: A physician with advanced training in a specific field to whom a patient is referred.

Speech and Language Pathologist: A person who is specially trained to diagnose, evaluate, and treat human communication problems and/or swallowing disorders.

Support Group: A group in which people with a common need or illness meet to share thoughts and feelings with others, and sometimes solve related problems.

Suppression: When disease symptoms recede or disappear while the patient is on medicine for that disease.

Symptoms: Evidence of a disease as perceived by the patient.

Syndrome: The symptoms of a disease perceived by a physician looking at the overall picture.

Systemic Lupus Erythematosus: A chronic auto-immune inflammatory disease with varied symptoms which affects connective tissue.

Therapy: The treatment of disease.

Tremor: Uncontrolled shaking in a part of the body.

Uremia: A condition characterized by insufficiently working kidneys, resulting in vomiting, nausea, an ammonia odor on the patient's breath, and sometimes causing the patient to lapse into a coma.

Vasculitis: Inflammation of the blood vessels.

Xerophthalmia: Dryness of the conjunctiva and cornea, as in Sjogren's Disease.

Xerostomia: Dryness in the mouth from lack of normal secretions, as in Sjogren's Disease.

BIBLIOGRAPHY

BOOKS

Adler, Joan. *The Retirement Book.* New York: William Morrow and Company, 1975.

Aladjem, Henrietta. *The Sun Is My Enemy: One Woman's Victory Over a Mysterious and Dreaded Disease (SLE).* Englewood Cliffs, N.J.: Prentice Hall, 1972.

Aladjem, Henrietta. *Lupus: Hope Through Understanding.* Lupus Foundation of America, 1982.

American Heart Association. *The American Heart Association Cookbook.* New York: David McKay Company, 1984.

American Medical Association. *The American Medical Association Book of Heart Care.* New York: Random House, 1982.

Ashton, Sherley. *How to Retire Successfully.* New York: Drake Publishers, 1977.

Benson, Herbert. *The Relaxation Response.* New York: Avon Books, 1976.

Berger, Gilda. *Physical Disabilities.* New York: Franklin Watts, 1979.

Bernheim, Kayla F.; Lewine, Richard R.J.; and Beale, Caroline T. *The Caring Family: Living with Chronic Mental Illness.* New York: Random House, 1982.

Berne, Eric, M.D. *Games People Play: The Psychology of Human Relationships.* New York: Grove Press, 1964.

Blau, Sheldon Paul, M.D., and Schultz, Dodi. *Lupus: The Body Against Itself.* Garden City, N.Y.: Doubleday and Company, 1978.

Bloomfield, Harold H., M.D.; Cain, Michael Peter; and Jafee, Dennis T. *TM: Discovering Inner Energy and Overcoming Stress.* New York: Delacorte Press, 1975.

Bowe, Frank. *Handicapping America: Barriers to Disabled People.* New York: Harper and Row, 1978.

Braverman, Jordan. *Crisis in Health Care.* Washington, D.C.: Acropolis Books Ltd., 1978.

Brena, S. F. *Chronic Pain: America's Hidden Epidemic.* New York: Atheneum/ SMI, 1978.

Brown, Robert N.; Allo, Clifford D.; Freeman, Alan D.; and Netzorg, Gordon W. *The Rights of Older Persons.* New York: Avon Books (American Civil Liberties Handbook), 1979.

Buckley, Joseph C. *The Retirement Handbook.* New York: Harper and Row, 1953.

Buscaglia, Leo. *The Disabled and Their Parents: A Counseling Challenge.* Thorofare N.J.: Charles B. Slack, Inc., 1975.

Butler, Robert N., M.D. *Why Survive? Being Old in America.* New York: Harper and Row, 1975.

Butler, Robert N., M.D., and Lewis, Myrna I. *Sex After Sixty: A Guide for Men and Women for Their Later Years.* New York: Harper and Row, 1976.

Cammer, Leonard. *Up From Depression.* New York: Simon and Schuster, 1969.

Comfort, Alex. *A Good Age.* New York: Crown Publishers, 1976.

Cousins, Norman. *Anatomy of an Illness as Perceived by the Patient.* New York: W.W. Norton and Company, 1979.

Eldridge, Priscilla B. *Caring for the Disabled Patient.* New Jersey: Litton Industries (Medical Economics Co.), 1978.

Fast, Julius. *Body Language.* New York: Simon and Schuster, 1970.

Fast, Julius. *Creative Coping: A Guide to Positive Living.* New York: William Morrow and Company, 1976.

Friedman, Jo-Ann. *Home Health Care: A Complete Guide for Patients and Their Families.* New York: W.W. Norton and Company, 1986.

Fries, James F., M.D., and Lorig, Kate. *Arthritis: A Comprehensive Guide.* Reading, Mass.: Addison-Wesley Publishing Company, 1980.

Galton, Lawrence. *The Disguised Disease: Anemia.* New York: Crown Publishers, 1975.

Gardner, A. W. *Dictionary of Symptoms: An Encyclopedic Guide to Medical Complaints, Symptoms and Terms.* New York: Gramercy Publishing Company, 1976.

Gaylin, Willard. *Caring.* New York: Alfred A. Knopf, 1976.

Gilbert, Sara. *Trouble at Home.* New York: Lothrop, Lee and Shepard Books, 1981.

Gillies, John. *A Guide to Caring for and Coping with Aging Parents.* Nashville: Thomas Nelson Publishers, 1981.

Ginott, Haim, M.D. *Between Parent and Child.* New York: Macmillan Company, 1965.

Ginott, Haim, M.D. *Between Parent and Teenager.* New York: Macmillan Company, 1969.

Goldberg, P., and Kaufman, D. *A Natural Sleep: How to Get Your Share.* Emmaus, Pa.: Rodale Press, 1978.

Granger, Stuart E. *Making Aids for Disabled Living.* London, England: B.T. Batsford, 1981.

Greenberg, Sidney. *A Treasury of Comfort.* New York: Crown Publishers, 1959.

Grollman, Earl L. *Concerning Death: A Practical Guide for the Living.* Boston: Beacon Press, 1974.

Halberstam, Michael, M.D., and Lesher, Stephan. *A Coronary Event.* Philadelphia: J.B. Lippincott Company, 1976.

Hale, G. *The Source Book for the Disabled.* New York: Paddington Press, 1979.

Haskins, James. *Who Are the Handicapped?* Garden City, N.Y.: Doubleday and Company, 1978.

Hendin, Herbert, M.D. *Suicide in America.* New York: W.W. Norton and Company, 1982.

Horowitz, Mardi J., M.D. *Stress Response Syndromes.* New York: Jason Aronson, Inc., 1976.

Inlander, Charles B., and Welner, Ed. *Take This Book to the Hospital with You.* Emmaus, Pa.: Rodale Press, 1985.

Institute of Rehabilitation Medicine. *Mealtime Manual for the Aged and Handicapped.* New York: Simon and Schuster (Essandess Special Edition), 1970.

Janov, Arthur. *Prisoners of Pain: Unlocking the Power of the Mind to End Suffering.* New York: Anchor Press, 1980.

Kaufman, Sherwin A. *Sexual Sabotage: How to Enjoy Sex in Spite of Physical and Emotional Problems.* New York: Macmillan Company, 1981.

Kerson, Toba Schwaber, and Kerson, Lawrence A. *Understanding Chronic Illness: The Medical and Psychosocial Dimensions of Nine Diseases.* New York: The Free Press, 1985.

Klinger, J. *Mealtime Manual for People with Disabilities and the Aging.* Camden, N.J.: Campbell Soup Company, 1978.

Knopf, Olga, M.D. *Successful Aging: The Facts and Fallacies of Growing Old.* New York: The Viking Press, 1975.

Krewer, Seymour. *The Arthritis Exercise Book.* New York: Simon and Schuster, 1981.

Kubler-Ross, Elisabeth. *Living With Death and Dying.* New York: Macmillan Company, 1981.

Kushner, Harold. *When All You've Ever Wanted Isn't Enough.* New York: Summit Books, 1986.

Kushner, Harold. *When Bad Things Happen to Good People.* New York: Avon Books, 1981.

Kutscher, Austin H., ed. *Death and Bereavement.* Springfield, Ill.: Charles C. Thomas Publishers, 1969.

Lagaala, B. *Caring for the Sick: Nursing the Ill, the Disabled, Children and the Elderly.* New York: Facts on File, 1982.

Lederer, Marculescu, Gallagher, and Mills. *Care Planning Pocket Guide: A Nursing Diagnostic Approach.* Menlo Park, Cal.: Addison-Wesley Publishing Company, 1986.

Lewis, Kathleen. *Successful Living with Chronic Illness.* Wayne, N.J.: Avery, 1985.

Lorig, Kate, and Fries, James F., M.D. *The Arthritis Helpbook.* Reading, Mass.: Addison-Wesley Publishing Company, 1980.

Mace, Nancy L. *The 36 Hour Day: A Family Guide to Caring for Persons with Alzheimer's Disease, Related Dementing Illnesses, and Memory Loss in Later Life.* Baltimore: Johns Hopkins University Press, 1981.

Maclay, Elise. *Green Winter: Celebrations of Old Age.* New York: Readers Digest Press, 1977.

Maltz, Maxwell, M.D. *Psycho-Cybernetics: A New Way to Get More Living Out of Life.* New York: Pb Special, 1966.

Masters, William H., and Johnson, Virginia E. *The Pleasure Bond: A New Look at Sexuality and Commitment.* Boston: Little, Brown and Company, 1970.

Masters, William H., and Johnson, Virginia E. *Human Sexual Response.* Boston: Little, Brown and Company, 1966.

May, Elizabeth Eckhardt; Waggoner, Neva R.; and Hotte, Eleanor Boettke. *Independent Living for the Handicapped.* Boston: Houghton Mifflin Company, 1974.

McCary, James Leslie. *Human Sexuality.* New York: Van Nostrand Reinhold Company, 1978.

McCollum, Audrey T. *The Chronically Ill Child: A Guide for Parents and Professionals.* Boston: Little, Brown and Company, 1981.

McConnell, Adeline, and Anderson, Beverly. *Single After Fifty: How to Have the Time of Your Life.* New York: McGraw Hill, 1981.

McQuade, Walter, and Aikman, Ann. *Stress: What it Is, What it Can Do to Your Health, How to Fight Back.* New York: E. P. Dutton and Co., Inc., 1974.

Melzack, Robert. *The Puzzle of Pain.* New York: Basic Books, 1973.

Melzack, Ronald, and Wall, Patricia D. *The Challenge of Pain.* New York: Basic Books, 1983.

Moos, Rudolf H., ed. *Coping With Physical Stress.* New York: Plenum Medical Book Company, 1977.

Nass, Terri, R.N. *Lupus Erythematosus: A Handbook for Nurses.* Milwaukee: 1984.

Nelson, James B. *Rediscovering the Person in Medical Care.* Minneapolis: Augsburg Publishing House, 1976.

Nuernberger, Phil. *Freedom from Stress: A Holistic Approach.* Honesdale, Pa.: Himalayan International Institute of Yoga Science and Philosophy Publishers, 1981.

Otten, Jane, and Shelley, Florence. *When Your Parents Grow Old.* New York: Funk and Wagnalls, 1976.

Papsidero, Joseph A.; Katz, Sidney, Sr.; Kroger, Mary Honora, R.S.M.; and Akpom, C. Amechi, eds. *Chance for a Change: Implications of a Chronic Disease Module Study.* East Lansing, Mich.: Michigan State University Press, 1979.

Park, Clara Clairborne, and Shapiro, Leon N. *You Are Not Alone: Understanding and Dealing with Mental Illness: A Guide for Patients, Families, Doctors and Other Professionals.* Boston: Little, Brown and Company, 1976.

Pease, Allan. *Signals: How to Use Body Language for Power, Success and Love.* New York: Bantam Books, 1984.

Pekkanen, John. *The Best Doctors in the U.S.* New York: Seaview Books, 1979.

Pelletier, K. *Mind as Healer, Mind as Slayer: A Holistic Approach to Preventing Stress Disorders.* Berkeley: Delacorte Press/Seymour Lawrence, 1976.

Pembrook, Linda. *How to Beat Fatigue.* Garden City, N.Y.: Doubleday and Company, 1976.

Phillips, Robert H. *Coping with Lupus.* Wayne, N.J.: Avery, 1984.

Raskas, Bernard S. *Heart of Wisdom, Book I.* New York: Burning Bush Press, 1962.

Raskas, Bernard S. *Heart of Wisdom, Book II.* New York: Burning Bush Press, 1979.

Raskas, Bernard S. *Heart of Wisdom, Book III.* New York: The United Synagogue Commission on Jewish Education, 1986.

Raskas, Bernard S. *Living Thoughts: Inspiration, Insight and Wisdom From Sources Throughout the Ages.* Bridgeport, Conn.: Hartmore House, 1976.

Reuben, David, M.D. *Everything You Always Wanted to Know About Sex.* New York: Bantam, 1969.

Rhodes, Sonya. *Surviving Family Life: The Seven Crises of Living Together.* New York: G.P. Putnam's Sons, 1981.

Robley, Spencer H. *Emphysema and Common Sense.* West Nyack, N.Y.: Parker Publishing Company, 1968.

Roth, Oscar, M.D. *Heart Attack: A Question and Answer Book.* Philadelphia, Pa.: J. B. Lippincott Company, 1978.

Rubin, Diane. *Caring: A Daughter's Story.* New York: Holt, Rinehart and Winston, 1982.

Sargent, Jean Vieth. *An Easier Way: Handbook for the Elderly and Handicapped.* Ames, Iowa: Iowa State University Press, 1984.

Sheehy, Gail. *Pathfinders.* New York: William Morrow and Company, 1981.

Silverstone, Barbara, and Hyman, Helen Kandell. *You and Your Aging Parent.* New York: Harper and Row, 1978.

Smolley, Bruce, M.D., and Schulman, Brian, M.D. *Pain Control: The Bethesda Program.* New York: Doubleday and Company, 1982.

Steward, Gordon W. *Every Body's Fitness Book.* New York: Dolphin, 1980.

Tavris, Carol. *Anger: The Misunderstood Emotion.* New York: Simon and Schuster, 1982.

Turk, Dennis C., and Kerns, Robert D. *Health, Illness, and Families: A Life-Span Perspective.* New York: Wiley-Interscience, 1985.

Veninga, Robert. *A Gift of Hope: How We Survive Our Strategies.* Boston: Little, Brown and Company, 1985.

Verby J., M.D., and Verby, J. *How to Talk to Your Doctors.* New York: Arco, 1977.

Vine, Phyllis. *Families in Pain: Children, Siblings, Spouses and Parents of the Mentally Ill Speak Out.* New York: Pantheon Books, 1982.

Viorst, Judith. *Necessary Losses: The Loves, Illusions, Dependencies and Impossible Expectations That All of Us Have to Give Up in Order to Grow.* New York: Simon and Schuster, 1986.

Weekes, Claire, M.D. *Hope and Help for Your Nerves.* New York: Hawthorne, 1969.

Wegscheider, Don. *If Only My Family Understood Me.* Minneapolis: Comp-Care Publications, 1979.

West, Charlene. *How to Live Single and Like It.* New York: Drake Publishers, 1977.

Whitbread, J. *Stop Hurting! Start Living! The Pain Control Book.* New York: Delacorte Press, 1981.

Zimmer, Arno B. *Employing the Handicapped: A Practical Compliance Manual.* New York: Amacon, 1981.

Zola, I. K. *Missing Pieces: A Chronicle of Living with a Disability.* Philadelphia, Pa.: Temple University Press, 1982.

PAMPHLETS AND BOOKLETS

American Heart Association. *Up and Around*. Dallas: 1979.

American Occupational Therapy Association, Inc., Practice Division. *Adapted Equipment*. Rockville, Md.

American Occupational Therapy Association, Inc., Division of Professional Development. *Handicapped Homemaker*. Rockville, Md.

Arthritis Foundation. *Arthritis, Living and Loving: Information About Sex*. Atlanta: 1982.

Arthritis Foundation. *Arthritis: The Basic Facts*. Atlanta: 1980.

Arthritis Foundation. *Home Care Programs in Arthritis*. Atlanta: 1980.

Arthritis Foundation. *So You Have . . . Osteoarthritis*. Atlanta: 1979.

Arthritis Foundation. *So You Have . . . Rheumatoid Arthritis*. Atlanta: 1981.

Anderson, Marion. *Occupational Lung Diseases*. The American Lung Association, 1983.

Barrett, Michael, Ph.D. *Sexuality and Multiple Sclerosis*. New York: National Multiple Sclerosis Society, 1982.

Burton, Charles, M.D., and Nida, Gail, R.N. *Be Good to Your Back*. Minneapolis: Sister Kenny Institute, 1980.

Carr, Ronald, M.D., Ph.D., and Jameson, Elizabeth. *Lupus Erythematosus: A Handbook for Physicians, Patients and their Families*. Lupus Foundation of America, 1982.

Channing L. Bete Company. *What Everyone Should Know About Asthma*. South Deerfield, Mass.: The American Lung Association, 1983.

Channing L. Bete Company. *What Everyone Should Know About Emphysema.* Greenfield, Mass.: The American Lung Association, 1976.

Dubois, Edmund L., M.D., and Cox, Mavis B. *Lupus Erythematosus.* Torrance, Cal.: The American Lupus Society, 1976.

Epstein, Wallace, M.D., and Clewley, Gina. *Living With S.L.E.: A Handbook for Patients With Systemic Lupus Erythematosus.* San Francisco: University of California, 1976.

Fowler, Roy S., Ph.D., and Fordyce, W.E., Ph.D. *Stroke: Why Do They Behave That Way?* Dallas: American Heart Association, 1981.

Harrower, Molly, Ph.D. *Mental Health and MS.* New York: National Multiple Sclerosis Society, 1979.

Haviland, Naomi; Kamil-Miller, Leslie; and Sliwa, Janet. *A Workbook for Consumers with Rheumatoid Arthritis.* University of Michigan Occupational Therapy Department, 1981.

Hogan, Sean. *Coping With Depression in a Chronic Illness.* From a speech at the Michigan Lupus Foundation, November 1977.

Jaffee, Cyrisse; Frankel, Debra; LaRache, Barbara; and Dick, Patricia. *Someone You Know Has Multiple Sclerosis: A Book for Families.* New York: National Multiple Sclerosis Society, 1982.

Le Maistre, JoAnn, Ph.D. *The Emotional Impact of Chronic Physical Disease.* Campbell, Cal.: Bay Area Lupus Foundation, Inc., 1981.

Liebling, Morton. *Spirit and Breath After Surgery: A Program on Rehabilitation by a Lung Cancer Patient.* Illinois.: American Cancer Society, 1979.

Lupus Foundation of America, Inc., Greater Atlanta Chapter. *Lupus Erythematosus,* Vol. 2 (1980), Vol. 3 (1982), Vol. 4 (1984). (Articles by physicians and medical professionals.)

Matson, Ronald R., and Brooks, Nancy A. *Adjusting to Multiple Sclerosis: An Exploratory Study.* National Multiple Sclerosis Society, 1981.

McGriff, Sylvia E. *Learning to Live With Neuromuscular Disease, A Message for Parents of Children with a Neuromuscular Disease.* New York: Muscular Dystrophy Association, 1981.

Muscular Dystrophy Association. *What Everyone Should Know About Muscular Dystrophy.* New York: 1981.

National Institutes of Health. *How to Cope With Arthritis.* Bethesda, Md.: October 1981.

National Institutes of Health, Office of Cancer Communications. *Taking Time—Support for People with Cancer and the People Who Care About Them.* Bethesda, Md.: 1982.

National Multiple Sclerosis Society. *Emotional Aspects of MS—Multiple Sclerosis.* New York: 1981.

Siegel, Irwin M., M.D. *Everybody's Different, Nobody's Perfect.* New York: Muscular Dystrophy Association, 1979.

U.S. Department of Health, Education, and Welfare. *Flexible Fashions: Clothing Tips for the Woman with Arthritis.* Pub. #1814, 1982.

MEDICAL JOURNAL ARTICLES

Banov, Charles H., M.D.; Buckley, Charles E., III, M.D.; Lockey, Richard F., M.D.; Rodriguez, Gilberto E., M.D.; Rosenthal, Richard R., M.D.; Harris, T. Reginald, M.D.; and Lothian, George G., M.D. "Confirming Asthma by Tests and Trials." *Patient Care*, August 15, 1981, pp. 31–52, 89–131.

Banov, Charles, H., M.D.; Buckley, Charles E., III, M.D.; Lockey, Richard F., M.D.; Rodriguez, Gilberto E., M.D.; Rosenthal, Richard R., M.D.; and Harris, T. Reginald, M.D. "Caring for the Patient with Asthma." *Patient Care*, August 15, 1981, pp. 25–27.

Bennerr, Robert M.; Bickel, Yale B.; Mack, Clayton L., M.D.; Goergen, Thomas G., M.D.; Wilske, Kenneth R., M.D.; and Reeves, James E., M.D. "When RA (Rheumatoid Arthritis) Requires Surgical Management." *Patient Care*, April 15, 1983, pp. 73–79.

Bogdan, Robert; Biklen, Douglas; Shapiro, Arthur; and Spelkoman, David. "The Disabled: Media's Monster." *Social Policy*, Fall 1982, pp. 32–35.

Bray, Grady P., Ph.D. "Sexual Function Poststroke." *Medical Aspects of Human Sexuality*, Vol. 18, No. 3. March 1984, pp. 115–123.

Brown, Julia S., Ph.D.; Rawlinson, May E., Ph.D.; and Hilles, Nancy, M. D. "Life Satisfaction and Chronic Disease, Exploration of a Theoretical Model." *Medical Care*, Vol. XIX, No. 11. November 1981, pp. 1136–1146.

Bruhn, John G., Ph.D. "Effect of Chronic Illness on the Family." *The Journal of Family Practice*, Vol. 4, No. 6. 1977, pp. 1057–1060.

Buchanan, Denton C., Ph.D. "Group Therapy for Chronic Physically Ill Patients." *Psychosomatics*, Vol. 19, No. 7. July 1978, pp. 425–431.

Chafetz, M.; Bernstein, N.; Sharpe, W.; and Schwab, R. "Short-Term Therapy of Patients with Parkinson's Disease." *The New England Journal of Medicine*, Vol. 253, No. 22. December 1, 1955.

Chopra, Sanjiv, M.D. (adapted from a lecture). "Extraintestinal Signs of Crohn's Disease." *Patient Care*, July 15, 1981, pp. 117–130.

Christopherson, Victor A., Ed.D. "Role Modification of the Handicapped Homemaker." *Rehabilitation Literature*, National Society for Crippled Children and Adults, Vol. 21, No. 4. April 1960.

Cluff, L. "Chronic Disease, Function and the Quality of Care." *Journal of Chronic Disease*, Vol. 34. 1981, pp. 299–304.

Cole, S.; O'Conner, S.; and Bennett, L. "Self Help Groups for Clinic Patients with Chronic Illness." *Primary Care*, Vol. 6, No. 2. June 1979.

Donabedian, Avedis, M.D., and Rosenfeld, Leonard S., M.D. "Follow-up Study of Chronically Ill Patients Discharged from Hospital." *Journal of Chronic Disease*, Vol. 17. 1964, pp. 847–862.

Dowling, John. "Autonomic Measures and Behavioral Indices of Pain Sensitivity." *Pain*, Vol. 16. 1983, pp. 193–200.

Falchuk, Z. Myron, M.D. (adapted from a lecture). "Crohn's Disease or Ulcerative Colitis?" *Patient Care*, July 15, 1981, pp. 105–114.

Freed, Murray M., M.D.; Kaplan, Lawrence I., M.D.; Klinger, Judith, OTR, MA; and Strebel, Miriam B., RN, OTR. "Improving Life for the Wheelchair User." *Patient Care*, June 15, 1984, pp. 48–86.

Gartner, Alan. "Images of the Disabled/Disabling Images." *Social Policy*, Fall 1982, pp. 14–15.

Hartings, M.; Pavlou, M.; and Davis, F. "Group Counseling of MS Patients in a Program of Comprehensive Care." *Journal of Chronic Diseases*, Vol. 29. 1976, pp. 65–73.

Kaplan, Robert M.; Atkins, Catherine J.; and Timms, Richard. "Validity of a Well-Being Scale as an Outcome Measure in Chronic Obstructive Pulmonary Disease." *Journal of Chronic Disease*, Vol. 37, No. 2. 1984, pp. 85–95.

Kimball, Chase P., M.D.; Kleeman, Charles R., M.D.; Rosenbaum, Ernest H., M.D.; Van Ven Noort, Stanley, M.D.; Wishner, William, J., M.D.; Murphy, Joseph P., M.D.; and Ganz, Richard, M.D. "Chronic Illness? Help the Family Cope." *Patient Care*, June 30, 1981, pp. 23–44.

Kimball, Chase P., M.D.; Kleeman, Charles R., M.D.; Rosenbaum, Ernest H., M.D.; Van Ven Noort, Stanley, M.D.; Wishner, William, J., M.D.; Murphy, Joseph P., M.D.; and Ganz, Richard, M.D. "Chronic Illness and Family Medicine." *Patient Care*, June 30, 1981, pp. 18–21.

Kinsman, Robert A., Ph.D.; Jones, Nelson F., Ph.D.; Matus, Irwin, Ph.D.; and Schum, Robert A., M.D. "Patient Variables Supporting Chronic Illness." *The Journal of Nervous and Mental Disease*, Vol. 163, No. 3. 1976, pp. 159–165.

Klein, R.; Dean, A.; and Bogdonoff, M. "The Impact of Illness Upon the Family." *Journal of Chronic Diseases*, Vol. 20. 1967, pp. 241–248.

Kravetz, Howard M., M.D., FCCP, and Pheatt, Nan, MPH. "Sexual Counseling for Pulmonary Patients." *Medical Aspects of Human Sexuality*, Vol. 18, No. 3. March 1984, pp. 146–161.

Kremer, Edwin F.; Atkinson, J. Hampton; and Kremer, Ann M. "The Language of Pain: Affective Descriptors of Pain are a Better Predictor of Psychological Disturbance than Pattern of Sensory and Affective Descriptors." *Pain*, Vol. 16. 1983, pp. 185–192.

Krupp, Neal E., M.D. "Adaptation to Chronic Illness." *Postgraduate Medicine*, Vol. 60, No. 5. November 1976, pp. 122–126.

Levy, Norman B., M.D. "The Chronically Ill Patient." *Psychiatric Quarterly*, Vol 51(3). Fall 1979, pp. 189–197.

Lipowski, Z.J., M.B., B.Ch. "Physical Illness, the Individual and the Coping Processes." *Psychiatry in Medicine*, Vol. 1. 1970, pp. 91–102.

Lisak, Robert P. "Myasthenia Gravis: Mechanisms and Management." *Hospital Practice*, March 1983, pp. 101–109.

Lockie, L. Maxwell; Gomez, Emoke; and Smith, Dennis M. "Low Dose Adrenocorticosteroids in the Management of Elderly Patients with Rheumatoid Arthritis: Selected Examples and Summary of Efficacy in the Long-Term Treatment of 97 Patients." *Seminars in Arthritis and Rheumatism*, Vol. 12, No. 4. May 1983, pp. 373–374.

Lowry, Michael R., and Atcherson, Esther. "Spouse-Assistants' Adjustment to Home Hemodialysis." *Journal of Chronic Disease*, Vol. 37, No. 4. 1984, pp. 293–300.

Mailick, M. "The Impact of Severe Illness on the Individual and Family: An Overview." *Social Work in Health Care*, Vol. 5(2). Winter 1979.

Miller, Frank, M.D. "Men Who Separate Love and Sex." *Medical Aspects of Human Sexuality*, Vol. 18, No. 3. March 1984, pp. 243–244.

"New Products." *Rehabilitation Literature*, Vol. 45, No. 3–4. March-April 1984, pp. 96–99.

Olsen, Edward H., M.D. "The Impact of Serious Illness on the Family System." *Post Graduate Medicine*, February 1970, pp. 169–174.

Pelachyk, John M.; Heinzerling, Rollin; and Burnham, Thomas K. "Serologic Profiles as Immunologic Markers for Different Clinical Presentations of Lupus Erythematosus." *Seminars in Arthritis and Rheumatism*, Vol. 12, No. 4. May 1983, pp. 382–389.

Quismorio, Francisco P., Jr.; Sharma, Om; Koss, Michael; Boylen, Thomas; Edmiston, Allen W.; Thornton, Phyllis J.; and Tatter, Dorothy. "Immunopathologic and Clinical Studies in Pulmonary Hypertension Associated with Systemic Lupus Erythematosus." *Seminars in Arthritis and Rheumatism*, Vol. 13, No. 4. May 1984, pp. 349–359.

Rusk, Howard A. "A Manual for Training the Disabled Homemaker." *Rehabilitation Monograph*, Institute of Rehabilitation Medicine, No. 3, Edition 2, 1961.

Starmer, C.; Lee, K.; Harrell, F.; and Rosati, R. "On the Complexity of Investigating Chronic Illness." *Biometrics*, Vol. 36. June 1980, pp. 333–335.

Strebel, Miriam Bowan, R.N., OTR, ed. "Adaptations and Techniques for the Disabled Homemaker." *Patient Care*, 5th edition. 1978.

Turk, Dennis, Ph.D.; Sobel, Harry J., Ph.D.; Follick, Michael, Ph.D; and Youkilis, Hildreth D., Ph.D. "A Sequential Criterion Analysis for Assessing Coping with Chronic Illness." *Journal of Human Stress*, June 1980, pp. 35–40.

Udelman, Harold D., M.D., and Udelman, Donna Lore, M.A. "The Family in Chronic Illness." *Arizona Medicine*, Vol. 37. 1980, pp. 491–493.

Vanderzwaag, R.; Mason, W.; Joyne, M.; and Runyan, J. "Cost of Chronic Disease Care." *Journal of Chronic Disease*, Vol. 33. 1980, pp. 713–720.

Viney, Linda L., and Westbrook, Mary T. "Coping with Chronic Illness: Strategy Preferences, Changes in Preferences and Associated Medical Reactions." *Journal of Chronic Disease*, Vol. 37, No. 6. 1984, pp. 489–502.

Wade, Charlotte, S., and Kramer, Roger M. "The Relationship Between Arthritic Adults and Furniture Usage: A Study." *Rehabilitation Literature*, Vol. 45, No. 3–4. March-April, 1984, pp. 80–84.

Zola, I. K. "Communication Barriers Between 'The Able-Bodied' and 'The Handicapped.'" *Archives of Physical Medicine Rehabilitation*, Vol. 62. August 1981.

INDEX

READER SURVEY

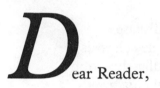ear Reader,

I want to write more about chronic illness. Your answers will help me decide what to write about next. It would help a great deal if you would take a few moments to fill out and mail this questionnaire.

If more than one person wants to fill out a questionnaire, please either make a copy or get additional copies from me (see address at the end of this survey). If you are willing to be included in follow-up studies, please be sure to include your name, address, and zip code at the end of this questionnaire. All responses are strictly confidential, and anonymous responses are okay.

Please send your completed Reader Survey to me at:

Sefra Pitzele
P.O. Box 16294
St. Paul, MN 55116

If more than one person wants to fill out a questionnaire, please either make a copy or get additional copies from me (see address at the end of this survey.) If you are willing to be included in follow-up studies, please be sure to include your name, address, and zip code at the end of this questionnaire.
Thank you for your help.

YOUR MEDICAL CONDITION

First, I'd like to get some basic information about your medical condition:

1. **What is your primary medical problem? Please check one. If you have two major medical problems, please number them 1 and 2 in order of severity (#1 as the most severe).**

    _____Alzheimer's disease   _____lung disease
    _____arthritis   _____multiple sclerosis
    _____asthma (severe, chronic)   _____muscular dystrophy
    _____cancer   _____myasthenia gravis
    _____diabetes   _____osteoarthritis
    _____discoid lupus   _____Parkinson's disease
    _____heart disease   _____result of accident or injury
    _____kidney disease   _____stroke impaired
    _____liver disease   _____systemic lupus
                                           erythematosus

    _____Other_____
    _____Don't have a chronic medical condition. I read this book for other reasons. (If this is the case, you may prefer to stop here.)

2. **How long have you been aware of your present medical condition?**

    _____less than 6 months   _____5 to 10 years
    _____6 months to 2 years   _____20 years or more
    _____2 to 5 years

3. **How long do you remember having symptoms before you first saw a doctor for your current problem?**

    _____no initial symptoms   _____6 to 12 months
    _____just a few weeks   _____between 1 and 5 years
    _____less than 6 months   _____more than 5 years

4. **Specifically, what were your symptoms?**

    _____

    _____

5. **How long did it take for a doctor to diagnose your medical condition?**
   _____just a few weeks   _____between 1 and 5 years
   _____less than 6 months   _____more than 5 years
   _____6 to 12 months

   5a. **Was the diagnosis made by your regular doctor?**
       _____ yes   _____ no

   5b. **If not, what kind of doctor diagnosed your condition?**

   _____

6. **Each person has unmet needs or frustrations. Do you have any unmet needs that are specific to your medical problem? (For example: "I can't get around in my apartment because it does not accommodate my wheelchair," "I have no one to talk to who really understands," "A physical barrier keeps me from getting around in my neighborhood," "My health insurance is inadequate and I can't keep up on my bills," or "I'd like to work but I can't.")**
   _____ yes   _____ no

   6a. **If yes, please list the three that are the most troublesome to you.**

   1. _____

   2. _____

   3. _____

7. **What resources in your community have helped you with your condition? (Example: Muscular Dystrophy Association, occupational therapy, special handicapped transportation programs.)**

   _____

   _____

YOU AND YOUR FAMILY

I'd like a better picture of you and your family, so I have a more complete picture of you.

8. **Are you:**
   _____ male   _____ female

9. **What was the last year of school that you completed?** _____

10. **What is your age?**
    _____under 25
    _____55 to 69
    _____25 to 39
    _____70 or older
    _____40 to 54

11. **Do any of your blood relatives also have a chronic illness?**
    _____ yes   _____ no

    11a. **If any blood relatives DO have a chronic illness, please make a check mark by each of the conditions below that applies.**

_____Alzheimer's disease	_____lung disease
_____arthritis	_____multiple sclerosis
_____asthma (severe, chronic)	_____muscular dystrophy
_____cancer	_____myasthenia gravis
_____diabetes	_____osteoarthritis
_____discoid lupus	_____Parkinson's disease
_____heart disease	_____result of accident or injury
_____kidney disease	_____stroke impaired
_____liver disease	_____systemic lupus erythematosus

    _____Other _____

12. **On a scale of 1–5, rate the quality of care you receive from your doctor. (For each item, 1 is very satisfied, 5 is dissatisfied.)**
    _____Physical (clinical) care

_____Treatment of conditions not related to my chronic condition
_____"Bedside manner"
_____Ongoing emotional support
_____Prompt response to phone calls
_____The credibility given to my symptoms
_____Uses language I understand to discuss my medical condition
_____Treats me courteously
_____Allows me to participate in my care
_____Other _____ (fill in)

12a. **If you are DISSATISFIED with some of the care you are receiving, what could your doctor do to improve?**

_____

_____

_____

13. **Have you seen medical specialists other than your regular doctor since your condition was diagnosed?**
_____ yes   _____ no

13a. **If yes, what kinds? (For example: cardiologist, kidney specialist, physical therapist, counselor, etc.)**

1. _____

2. _____

3. _____

14. **About how often do you see your regular doctor primarily regarding your chronic medical condition?**
_____once a week   _____once a year
_____once a month   _____less than once a year
_____twice a year

14a. **Do you feel your chronic disease keeps you from having regular physicals?**

14b. **If so, why?** _____

RELATIONSHIPS

A chronic medical condition will often affect marriage and family relationships. I would appreciate any information you can give me which will help me understand these issues better.

15. **What is your present marital status?**
    _____single, never married   _____divorced
    _____married   _____widowed
    _____married, but separated

16. **Were you married when your condition was diagnosed?**
    _____ yes   _____ no

17. **If you were divorced or separated AFTER your medical condition was diagnosed, do you feel your medical condition was in any way responsible?**
    _____ yes   _____ no

17a. **If yes, please explain.**

    1. _____

    2. _____

    3. _____

18. **Have you become involved in a romantic relationship since your medical condition developed?**
    _____ yes   _____ no

18a. **Do you feel that your medical condition is a barrier to close emotional ties with others?**
_____yes, definitely
_____yes, to some degree
_____no

WORK

Chronic medical conditions may change how much you can work, where you work, and what kind of job you can do. I'd like to get some information about your work.

19. **Were you working outside of your home at the time of your diagnosis?**
_____ yes   _____ no

20. **Are you currently working?**
_____ yes   _____ no

21. **If you are NOT currently working:**

21a. **Have you ever worked?**
_____ yes   _____ no

21b. **If you have stopped working, what was the primary reason?**
_____My disability is too severe
_____I am on a disability pension
_____I am being re-trained
_____I am retired
_____I don't wish to work (unrelated to my chronic condition)
_____I can't find a job
_____I am in school
_____Other: _____

22. **If you ARE currently working:**

22a. **Are you working full time or part time?**
_____ full time   _____ part time

22b. **Are you the primary wage earner in your household?**

_____yes   _____no

I contribute ____% of the income

22c. **Are you working at the same job as you were when you were first diagnosed?**

_____ yes   _____ no

22d. **Has your medical condition caused you to change jobs?**

_____ yes   _____ no

If yes, what change have you made?

I used to work as a _____

Now I work as a _____

23. **If you are currently working or have worked since your medical condition developed:**

23a. **Have you reduced your number of working hours because of your condition?**

_____ yes   _____ no

23b. **Were there/Are there any physical changes made at your place of employment to accommodate your special needs?**

_____ yes   _____ no

If yes, please describe them:

_____

_____

_____

23c. **Has your employer permitted you to take the rest breaks you've needed?**

_____yes, usually

_____yes, sometimes

_____no, never/rarely

_____I have not needed rest breaks

YOUR LIVING SITUATION

I'd like to know about any changes that your medical condition has caused you to make in the place where you live.

24. **Did you have to make any changes in you living place to accommodate your medical condition?**

_____ yes   _____ no

24a. **If yes, what, specifically, did you have to change?** (Please describe the change in the space provided after each item.)

____Kitchen _____

_____

____Living room _____

_____

____Bedroom _____

_____

____Bathroom _____

_____

_____Eating area _____

_____

_____Garage _____

_____

_____Car _____

_____

_____Exterior (stairs, walk, etc.) _____

_____

_____Have had to move to another living situation. Please explain:

_____

_____Other _____

INSURANCE

A chronic medical condition often causes financial problems. Your health becomes a major concern and insurance may become hard to get. Please give me some information about your insurance.

25. **Did you have any health insurance when your medical condition developed?**
     _____ yes   _____ no

   25a. **Do you have any kind of health insurance NOW?**
         _____ yes   _____ no

25b. **If yes, what kinds? Please include health maintenance organizations (HMO's), Veteran's Administration Assistance, Medicaid, and Medicare if they apply.**

_____

_____

26. **Have your premiums increased as a result of your medical condition?**
_____ yes   _____ no

26a. **If yes, please state why, specifically.**

_____

_____

_____

27. **Have you ever had your insurance cancelled because of your medical condition?**
_____ yes   _____ no

SUPPORT GROUPS

A chronic medical condition can cause many changes in your personal life and in your work. Many people find help in support groups. Please tell me about your experiences, if any, with these groups:

28. **Do you belong to any kind of group that helps you deal with and learn about your condition?**
_____ yes   _____ no

29. **If you do NOT belong to a group, it is because (check all that apply):**
_____ I don't know where to go   _____ I don't feel I need it
_____ There isn't one nearby   _____ Other _____

30. **If you DO belong to a group, do you find it helpful?**
   _____ yes   _____ no

   30a. **What organization sponsors the program?**

   _____

   30b. **How often does the group meet?** _____

   30c. **What types of group activities are most helpful to you?** (For example: a speaker, seminars, talking with others, etc.)

   _____

THIS BOOK AND THE AUTHOR

I need feedback, too.

31. **Do you feel that you benefited by reading WE ARE NOT ALONE?**
   _____ yes   _____ no   _____ somewhat

32. **If you feel you did benefit in some way, please check the chapters you found most helpful. Then, if you can, describe more specifically what it was that helped you.**

   _____Chapter 1: Who promised life would always be fair?

   _____

   _____Chapter 2: First, there is the diagnosis

   _____

   _____Chapter 3: Grieving is normal

   _____

____Chapter 4: In sickness and in health

_____

____Chapter 5: But who will take me to the zoo?

_____

____Chapter 6: Keeping up your friendships

_____

____Chapter 7: Partners in your health care team

_____

____Chapter 8: The circle of stress, illness, and pain

_____

____Chapter 9: Comments on depression

_____

____Chapter 10: Blessed are the caregivers

_____

____Chapter 11: Resting, relaxing, and related concerns

_____

____Chapter 12: A whisper in the night

_____

_____Chapter 13: Bodywork

_____

_____Chapter 14: Adaptive living strategies

_____

_____Chapter 15: Practical matters

_____

33. **If you could add anything to make this a better book, what would you add?**

_____

_____

_____

Thank you for your participation.

If you have suggestions you want to pass along to others in your situation, or if you need another copy of this Reader Survey, please write me at:

Sefra Korbin Pitzele
P.O. Box 16294
St. Paul, MN 55116

OPTIONAL: If you wish to be included in further needs assessments or surveys, please include your name, address and zip code. Be assured that your name and address will go no further than my desk drawer; they will only be used to mail you new surveys.

Name:_____

Address:_____

City, State, and Zip Code_____